AF377757

Morphological and Biochemical Characterization of Aerobic and Anaerobic Bacteria

Morphological and Biochemical Characterization of Aerobic and Anaerobic Bacteria

Dr. Hariharan AG

M. Pharm, PhD

Dr. Neelesh Malviya

M. Pharm, PhD

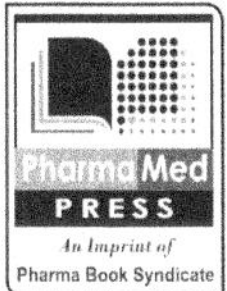

PharmaMed Press

An imprint of Pharma Book Syndicate

A unit of BSP Books Pvt. Ltd.

4-4-309/316, Giriraj Lane,

Sultan Bazar, Hyderabad - 500 095.

Morphological and Biochemical Characterization of Aerobic and Anaerobic Bacteria *by* Hariharan AG and Neelesh Malviya

Published by

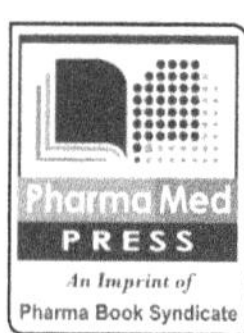

PharmaMed Press

An imprint of Pharma Book Syndicate

A unit of BSP Books Pvt. Ltd.
4-4-309/316, Giriraj Lane, Sultan Bazar, Hyderabad - 500 095.
Phone: 040-23445688, 23445600; Fax: 91+40-23445611
E-mail: info@pharmamedpress.com
www.pharmamedpress.com/pharmamedpress.net

ISBN: 978-93-88305-93-8

PREFACE

The Human race has always played distinguished attention in exploring the knowledge on various aspects of the materials present in this planet. The contribution of Louis Pasteur (1822-1895), Robert Koch (1843-1910) and many other scientists had helped us in gathering the knowledge about microbiology.

This practical guide had prepared with the objective to explain the most basic techniques used in general microbiology. Mastering these methods will help the students to apply the techniques of aseptic work, sterilization and disinfection, or work with laboratory cultures.

The series of practical exercises has been designed and compiled mainly according to the logic of the exploration and description of the microbial diversity of an environment. Thus, it starts with the description of a microbiological laboratory especially about the various Bio safety levels, preparatory work such as Media preparations and its sterilization, etc., environmental sampling.

The main focus was on the characterization of bacteria especially the Morphological characterization like microscopic investigation of by various staining techniques and the Biochemical characterization, which effectively help in the identification of particular strain of both aerobic and anaerobic bacteria.

This book also covers some important aspects for the pharmaceutical student's especially in the understating of the Assay of Antibiotics and Sterility testing.

This book has been written in simple language, easily understandable for the students who can easily perform the practical exercise helps in systematized characterization of microorganism. This book would be useful for students of Medical sciences and Paramedical sciences of certificate and graduate levels such as B.Pharm, Certificate Nursing, Laboratory Technician, Health Assistant, B. Sc Nursing, Bachelor of Nursing (B N), B. Sc Medical Microbiology, Bachelor in Medical Laboratory Technologist (BMLT), B. Sc Microbiology, Bachelor in Public Health (BPH), Bachelor in Dental Surgery (BDS), Bachelor in Medicine and Bachelor in Surgery (MBBS).

Numerous references have been consulted in preparation of this book and I thank the many investigators whose findings I have drawn upon so heavily. I apologize for any kind of mistakes or errors in this book. I am grateful to my Guru (Teachers), my collogues and my family members for their valuable suggestions, constant encouragement and support. I warmly welcome the critical comments and suggestions from Professors, Teachers, Consultant microbiologist, Students and other readers. Their valuable suggestions will be given due consideration in the next edition.

- Authors

CONTENTS

PART V

PART VI

PART VII

PART VIII

PART - I
INTRODUCTION TO MICROBIOLOGY

Chapter 1

History of Microbiology

Microbiology

Microbiology is a Greek term meaning micro = small, Bio = life, and logos = discourse or study. In a broader way it can be defined as the science or study of microscopic organisms which includes virus, bacteria, fungi algae and protozoa (have microscopic stages during their life cycles) and some play a role in disease transmission. Humans have been interacting with microorganisms for thousands of years but their significance was appreciated only 200 years before. Today microbiology is recognized as a subject of major importance since it plays a major role in nearly every aspect of our lives. Microbiology encompasses numerous sub-disciplines like virology, mycology, parasitology, bacteriology etc. The microbiology had been applied in various fields

1. **Medical microbiology:** The study of the pathogenic microbes and the role of microbes in human diseases and its epidemiology and it also include the study of disease pathology and immunology.

2. **Pharmaceutical microbiology:** The study of microorganisms that are related to the production of antibiotics, enzymes, vitamins, vaccines, and other pharmaceutical products and that cause pharmaceutical contamination and spoil.

3. **Industrial microbiology:** The exploitation of microbes for use in industrial processes like industrial fermentation and wastewater treatment.

4. **Microbial biotechnology:** The manipulation of microorganisms at the genetic and molecular level to generate useful products.

5. **Food microbiology and Dairy microbiology:** The study of microorganisms causing food spoilage and foodborne illness. Using microorganisms to produce foods, for example by fermentation.

6. **Agricultural microbiology:** The study of agriculturally relevant microorganisms like the study of the interactions between

microorganisms and plants and plant pathogens, study of those microorganisms that are found in soil.

7. **Veterinary microbiology:** The study of the role of microbes in veterinary medicine or animal taxonomy.

8. **Environmental microbiology:** The study of the function and diversity of microbes in their natural environments. This involves the characterization of key bacterial habitats such as the rhizosphere and phyllosphere, soil and groundwater ecosystems, open oceans or extreme environments (extremophiles).

History of Microbiology

Evolution: Single-celled microorganisms were the first forms of life to develop on Earth, approximately 3–4 billion years ago. Bacteria, algae and fungi have been identified in amber that is 220 million years old, which shows that the morphology of microorganisms has changed little since the Triassic period.

Infectious Disease: Bubonic plague is the first known epidemic caused by microorganism *Yersinia pestis (formerly known as Pasteurella pestis)* is believed to be the cause of the Black Death that swept through Europe in the 14th century and killed an estimated 25 million people, or 30–60% of the European population.

The first cholera pandemic (1819–24), also known as the first Asiatic cholera pandemic or Asiatic cholera, began near Calcutta and spread throughout Southeast Asia to the Middle East, eastern Africa and the Mediterranean coast. Hundreds of thousands of people died as a result of this pandemic, including many British soldiers, which attracted European attention.

Beverages: Apart from evolution and disease, prior to 6000 BC human societies Sumerians and Babylonians were started using micro-organisms to ferment grain and make beer. Alcoholic beverages made from rice were produced in China as early as 2300 BC. Around 4000 BC the Egyptians discovered that bread dough treated in a certain manner, would rise into a light airy loaf.

Invention of Microscope

Anton Van Leeuwenhoek (1674-1676)

The discovery of microbiology is usually credited to a Dutch naturalist by the name of Anton Van Leeuwenhoek. He ground fine glass lenses (which could magnify objects about 266 times) and observed living microorganisms (which he called "animalcules") from a variety of environments. He documented his findings and sent correspondence to the British Royal Society or Royal Society of London in 1684, and thereby aroused considerable interest in microbiology.

Development of Microbiology

Spontaneous Generation (Abiogenesis)

Van Leeuwenhoek's discoveries did much to revitalize arguments between scientists, philosophers and theologians about the origin of life. Theory of **abiogenesis** or **spontaneous generation** (a=without, bio=life, genesis=origins or beginnings) was taught by Aristotle around 346 BC. He believed that life could and did appear spontaneously from non-living and/or decomposing materials. For example, he wrote that snakes and frogs came from the mud along river banks.

Around 1665 the Italian naturalist and physician **Francesco Redi** demonstrated that spontaneous generation did not occur at a macroscopic level using flies. Redi placed raw meat into containers and covered some with gauze and some with paper. Other containers were left open. He found that the meat within the covered containers did not develop flies, but that flies did lay eggs on the gauze and on the paper. The exposed meat developed maggots, but he reasoned that these came from the eggs of flies, not from the meat itself. Regardless of Redi's proof, people still clung to their belief in abiogenesis, and Van Leeuwenhoek's discoveries seemed to support this theory.

In 1749, John Needham, a Catholic priest, conducted experiments with mutton broth in flasks. He boiled the broth and stoppered the flasks with cork, but later found the broth to be teaming with microorganisms. Needham believed there was a "vital force" present within the broth, and that life had arisen spontaneously.

In 1766, **Lazzaro Spallanzani**, a priest by profession but scientist at heart, repeated Needham's experiments. Spallanzani boiled his broth longer and sealed his flasks with glass. After several days the flasks were opened and were found to contain no living organisms. Needham and others discredited Spallanzani's work because they said his prolonged boiling had destroyed the "vital force" within the broth, and because no air could get in. (The discovery of oxygen and its importance to life had occurred at about the same time.) Thus, although Spallanzani had actually proven that microorganisms did not arise spontaneously from non-living materials, he was not credited for his work at the time.

During the 1830s, Theodor Schwann and Franz Schultz (both German scientists) conducted experiments to disprove abiogenesis. They allowed boiled broth to come into contact with air that was either heated or passed through solutions of toxic chemicals. No microscopic organisms grew in their broth. Again the "vitalists", those in favor of spontaneous generation, discredited this work because they said the drastic treatment of the air had rendered it inactive.

Louis Pasteur (1860s), constructed "goose necked" flasks, in which he could boil nutrient broths but their shape, prevented the entrance of microorganisms from air. Though these were left open to whatever "vital forces" might be present in air, no organisms grew. Fortunately, Pasteur's broths contained no endospore forming bacteria, since endospores are resistant to boiling and had they been present, would have grown. Though Pasteur's work was not universally accepted, he had many supporters. Though many investigators worked to disprove the theory of abiogenesis at the microscopic level, it is Pasteur who usually receives credit for finally laying the theory to rest. Once this was accomplished, the supernatural, mysterious or magical aspects of microorganisms were explained away, and Microbiology could be recognized as a true science.

Germ Theory of Disease

Hypocrites believed that people could transmit disease from one to another, but they did not understand how. Around 1546, **Girolamo Fracastoro**, an Italian physician, recorded his belief that disease was due to organisms too small to be seen with the naked eye. This was referred to as the contagion theory, but since Fracastoro had no real proof, his writings were largely ignored. Since people were unaware of disease causing microbes and their manner of transmission, practices we take for granted today (to prevent infection and contamination) did not occur to people.

Robert Koch (1876)

In 1867 Robert Koch, a German physician had provided direct evidence demonstrating that bacteria were disease-causing agents. Koch was working with anthrax; a disease of sheep and cattle and determined the causative agent to be a bacterium *Bacillus anthracis*. Koch established a sequence of experimental steps that could be used to demonstrate beyond a doubt that a specific type of microorganism was responsible for a specific disease. These came to be known as **Koch's postulates**, and are still in use today.

Koch's Postulates

1. The suspect causative agent must be found in every case of the disease. (Koch took samples from hundreds of animals over years of investigation to be certain of his conclusions.)

2. The specific type of microbe must be isolated from the infected individual and grown in a culture containing no other forms (pure culture).

3. Upon inoculation into a normal, healthy, susceptible animal, a pure culture of the microbial agent must produce the disease.

4. The same type of microbe must be recovered again from the experimentally infected host.

Fortunately for Koch, he was working with a relatively large and easily cultured type of microorganism. His postulates are applicable only if the microorganisms associated with a particular disease can be isolated and grown in an artificial environment, and for some types of microbes, this is much more difficult. Because of Koch's work, the etiological agents for many important human diseases were identified in rapid succession between the years of 1876 and 1898. By 1900, the microorganisms responsible for major human diseases including cholera, diphtheria, leprosy, plague, tetanus, tuberculosis and typhoid had been identified. The period of years between 1857 and 1914 is sometimes referred to as the "Golden Age of Microbiology", because rapid advancements and discoveries made during this period led to the establishment of microbiology as a science. During their search for disease causing agents, Koch and other microbiologists made important contributions to the techniques and materials used in the culture of microorganisms. Some of these important developments involved the following people.

Richard J. Petri - developed the **Petri dish** in which microbial cultures could be grown and manipulated.

Fanny Hesse - developed the use of **agar** as a solidifying agent for microbiological media.

Hans Christian Gram - developed the **Gram stain**, a stain technique that could be used to separate two major groups of disease causing bacteria.

Discovery of Disinfectant

Joseph Lister (1867)

During the 1860s **Joseph Lister**, an English surgeon reasoned that surgical infection might be caused by microorganisms. Lister devised methods to prevent microbes from entering the wounds of his patients. His procedures came to be known as **antiseptic** (against sepsis) surgery, and included hand washing, sterilizing instruments, and dressing wounds with carbolic acid (phenol). These techniques also provided indirect evidence for the connection between micro-organisms and disease.

Immunization

In 1796, **Edward Jenner** (a British Physician) reported the use of material scraped from the skin of an individual infected with cowpox to immunize a child against smallpox. Jenner had noticed that dairymaids (young women responsible for milking cows) frequently contracted cowpox, a relatively mild disease, but were resistant to smallpox. Since both of these diseases are caused by viruses, there was no way for Jenner to see the disease causing agents, but his method was successful. He called his technique **vaccination** (vacca = cow).

In 1880, **Louis Pasteur** had isolated the bacteria responsible for causing chicken cholera (organisms similar to the ***Vibrio cholerae*** causing cholera in humans). He later arranged for a public demonstration of Koch's postulates and inoculated a number of animals with the pure culture he had prepared. Much to his dismay, the animals did not develop disease symptoms, but remained perfectly healthy. Upon reviewing his records, Pasteur found that the experimental animals had been inoculated with a culture several weeks old. Pasteur reasoned that this old culture would be weakened (**attenuated**) and might therefore be unable to cause disease. He arranged to repeat the demonstration, and this time inoculated the subject animals with a fresh culture. Fortunately he also chose to inoculate a new group of animals with the same culture. The original animals again did not develop disease symptoms, but the newly inoculated animals did. As expected, they all developed cholera and died. Pasteur knew that the experimental animals had all been inoculated with the same type of disease causing bacteria. Since they all came from a similar source, he suspected that exposure to the attenuated culture had somehow made the first ones resistant to the disease. He repeated the experiments and eventually concluded that this was indeed the case. Bacteria that were killed or attenuated could be used to prevent disease. Pasteur called his attenuated cultures **vaccines**, and thus gave credit to an earlier investigator named Edward Jenner.

Future of Microbiology

By the early 1900s, physicians knew that microorganisms could cause disease, and under certain circumstances could be used to prevent disease, but they did not know how to cure disease. Many strange and sometimes brutal practices had been used in attempts to cure disease, but most were useless and some were dangerous (for example the ingestion of precious metals - gold and silver). What was needed was substances that could be taken into the body and would somehow seek out and kill the pathogenic microorganisms without harming the patient, i.e., a "magic bullet".

A German physician by the name of **Paul Ehrlich** searched for a "magic bullet", and in around 1910 developed the first effective cure for a bacterial disease. The drug he developed was called **salvarsan**, and was an arsenic compound that was effective against syphilis. A short time later (1928), **Alexander Fleming**, a Scottish physician, discovered penicillin. He had noticed that a mold growing on one of his culture plates inhibited the growth of bacteria there, and eventually isolated the substance responsible. Penicillin was among the first antibiotics to be used in the treatment of disease.

During the 20th century, microbiology has expanded and increased in importance. Immunology, virology and molecular genetics (recombinant DNA technology) have arisen as branches of microbiology. New discoveries in microbiology may lead to better methods for food and fuel production as well as environmental remediation that will become more and more critical as the human population continues to expand. Or perhaps microbes will eventually force humans to live in balance with the natural world.

Modern microbiology reaches into many fields of human endeavor, including the development of pharmaceutical products, the use of quality-control methods in food and dairy product production, the control of disease-causing microorganisms in consumable waters, and the industrial applications of microorganisms. Microorganisms are used to produce vitamins, amino acids, enzymes, and growth supplements. They manufacture many foods, including fermented dairy products (sour cream, yogurt, and buttermilk), as well as other fermented foods such as pickles, sauerkraut, breads, and alcoholic beverages.

Over the past four decades, *Biosafety in Microbiological and Biomedical Laboratories* (BMBL) has become the code of practice for biosafety in US (the discipline addressing the safe handling and containment of infectious microorganisms and hazardous biological materials). The principles of biosafety were introduced in 1984 to understand the containment and risk assessment.

- The fundamental of containment includes the microbiological practices, safety equipment, and facility safeguards that protect laboratory workers, the environment, and the public from exposure to infectious microorganisms that are handled and stored in the laboratory.

- Risk assessment is the process that enables the appropriate selection of microbiological practices, safety equipment, and facility safeguards that can prevent laboratory-associated infections (LAI).

The four ascending levels of containment, referred to as biosafety levels 1 through 4, are infectivity, severity of disease, transmissibility, and the nature of the work being conducted. Another important risk factor for agents that cause moderate to severe disease is the origin of the agent, whether indigenous or exotic. Each level of containment describes the microbiological practices, safety equipment and facility safeguards for the corresponding level of risk associated with handling of a particular agent. The basic practices and equipment are appropriate for protocols common to most research and clinical laboratories. The facility safeguards help protect non-laboratory occupants of the building and the public health and environment (Table 1.1).

1. **Biosafety level 1 (BSL-1)** is the basic level of protection and is appropriate for agents that are not known to cause disease in normal, healthy humans.

2. **Biosafety level 2 (BSL-2)** is appropriate for handling moderate-risk agents that cause human disease of varying severity by ingestion or through percutaneous or mucous membrane exposure.

3. **Biosafety level 3 (BSL-3)** is appropriate for agents with a known potential for aerosol transmission, for agents that may cause serious and potentially lethal infections and that are indigenous or exotic in origin.

4. **Biosafety level 4 (BSL-4)** Exotic agents that pose a high individual risk of life threatening disease by infectious aerosols and for which no treatment is available are restricted to high containment laboratories that meet biosafety level 4 (BSL-4) standards.

Biosafety Level 1

Biosafety Level 1 is suitable for work involving well-characterized agents not known to consistently cause disease in immunocompetent adult humans, and present minimal potential hazard to laboratory personnel and the environment. BSL-1 laboratories are not necessarily separated from the general traffic patterns in the building. Work is typically conducted on open bench tops using standard microbiological practices. Special containment equipment or facility design is not required, but may be used as determined by appropriate risk assessment. Laboratory personnel must have specific training in the procedures conducted in the laboratory and must be supervised by a scientist with training in microbiology or a related science.

The following standard practices, safety equipment, and facility requirements apply to BSL-1:

A. Standard Microbiological Practices

1. The laboratory supervisor must enforce the institutional policies that control access to the laboratory.

2. Persons must wash their hands after working with potentially hazardous materials and before leaving the laboratory.

3. Eating, drinking, smoking, handling contact lenses, applying cosmetics, and storing food for human consumption must not be permitted in laboratory areas. Food must be stored outside the laboratory area in cabinets or refrigerators designated and used for this purpose.

4. Mouth pipetting is prohibited; mechanical pipetting devices must be used.

5. Policies for the safe handling of sharps, such as needles, scalpels, pipettes, and broken glassware must be developed and implemented. Whenever practical, Laboratory supervisors

should adopt improved engineering and work practice controls that reduce risk of sharps injuries.

Precautions, including those listed below, must always be taken with sharp items. These include:

(a) Careful management of needles and other sharps are of primary importance. Needles must not be bent, sheared, broken, recapped, removed from disposable syringes, or otherwise manipulated by hand before disposal.

(b) Used disposable needles and syringes must be carefully placed in conveniently located puncture-resistant containers used for sharps disposal.

(c) Non disposable sharps must be placed in a hard walled container for transport to a processing area for decontamination, preferably by autoclaving.

(d) Broken glassware must not be handled directly. Instead, it must be removed using a brush and dustpan, tongs, or forceps. Plastic-ware should be substituted for glassware whenever possible.

(e) Perform all procedures to minimize the creation of splashes and/or aerosols.

(f) Decontaminate work surfaces after completion of work and after any spill or splash of potentially infectious material with appropriate disinfectant.

(g) Decontaminate all cultures, stocks, and other potentially infectious materials before disposal using an effective method. Depending on where the decontamination will be performed, the following methods should be used prior to transport:

(i) Materials to be decontaminated outside of the immediate laboratory must be placed in a durable, leak proof container and secured for transport.

(ii) Materials to be removed from the facility for decontamination must be packed in accordance with applicable local, state, and federal regulations.

(h) A sign incorporating the universal biohazard symbol must be posted at the entrance to the laboratory when infectious agents are present. The sign may include the name of the agent(s) in use, and the name and phone number of the laboratory supervisor or other responsible personnel. Agent information should be posted in accordance with the institutional policy.

(i) An effective integrated pest management program is required.

(j) The laboratory supervisor must ensure that laboratory personnel receive appropriate training regarding their duties, the necessary precautions to prevent exposures, and exposure evaluation procedures. Personnel must receive annual updates or additional training when procedural or policy changes occur. Personal health status may impact an individual's susceptibility to infection, ability to receive immunizations or prophylactic interventions. Therefore, all laboratory personnel and particularly women of child-bearing age should be provided with information regarding immune competence and conditions that may predispose them to infection. Individuals having these conditions should be encouraged to self-identify to the institution's healthcare provider for appropriate counseling and guidance.

B. Special Practices

None required.

C. Safety Equipment (Primary Barriers and Personal Protective Equipment)

1. Special containment devices or equipment, such as Bio Safety Cabinets (BSCs) not generally required.

2. Protective laboratory coats, gowns, or uniforms are recommended to prevent contamination of personal clothing.

3. Wear protective eyewear when conducting procedures that have the potential to create splashes of microorganisms or other hazardous materials. Persons who wear contact lenses in laboratories should also wear eye protection.

4. Gloves must be worn to protect hands from exposure to hazardous materials. Glove selection should be based on an appropriate risk assessment. Alternatives to latex gloves should be available. Wash hands prior to leaving the laboratory. In addition, BSL-1 workers should:

    (a) Change gloves when contaminated, integrity has been compromised, or when otherwise necessary.

    (b) Remove gloves and wash hands when work with hazardous materials has been completed and before leaving the laboratory.

    (c) Do not wash or reuse disposable gloves. Dispose off used gloves with other contaminated laboratory waste. Hand washing protocols must be rigorously followed.

D. Laboratory Facilities (Secondary Barriers)

(a) Laboratories should have doors for access control.

(b) Laboratories must have a sink for hand washing.

(c) The laboratory should be designed so that it can be easily cleaned. Carpets and rugs in laboratories are not appropriate.

(d) Laboratory furniture must be capable of supporting anticipated loads and uses. Spaces between benches, cabinets, and equipment should be accessible for cleaning.

  (i) Bench tops must be impervious to water and resistant to heat, organic solvents, acids, alkalis, and other chemicals.

  (ii) Chairs used in laboratory work must be covered with a non-porous material that can be easily cleaned and decontaminated with appropriate disinfectant.

(e) Laboratories windows that open to the exterior should be fitted with screens.

Biosafety Level 2

Biosafety Level 2 builds upon BSL-1. BSL-2 is suitable for work involving agents that pose moderate hazards to personnel and the environment. It differs from BSL-1 in that

1. Laboratory personnel have specific training in handling pathogenic agents and are supervised by scientists competent in handling infectious agents and associated procedures.

2. Access to the laboratory is restricted when work is being conducted.

3. All procedures in which infectious aerosols or splashes may be created are conducted in BSCs or other physical containment equipment.

4. The following standard and special practices, safety equipment, and facility requirements apply to BSL-2:

A. Standard Microbiological Practices

1. The laboratory supervisor must enforce the institutional policies that control access to the laboratory.

2. Persons must wash their hands after working with potentially hazardous materials and before leaving the laboratory.

3. Eating, drinking, smoking, handling contact lenses, applying cosmetics, and storing food for human consumption must not be permitted in laboratory areas. Food must be stored outside

the laboratory area in cabinets or refrigerators designated and used for this purpose.

4. Mouth pipetting is prohibited; mechanical pipetting devices must be used.

5. Policies for the safe handling of sharps, such as needles, scalpels, pipettes, and broken glassware must be developed and implemented. Whenever practical, laboratory supervisors should adopt improved engineering and work practice controls that reduce risk of sharps injuries.

Precautions, including those listed below, must always be taken with sharp items. These include:

(a) Careful management of needles and other sharps are of primary importance. Needles must not be bent, sheared, broken, recapped, removed from disposable syringes, or otherwise manipulated by hand before disposal.

(b) Used disposable needles and syringes must be carefully placed in conveniently located puncture-resistant containers used for sharps disposal.

(c) Non-disposable sharps must be placed in a hard walled container for transport to a processing area for decontamination, preferably by autoclaving.

(d) Broken glassware must not be handled directly. Instead, it must be removed using a brush and dustpan, tongs, or forceps. Plastic-ware should be substituted for glassware whenever possible.

1. Perform all procedures to minimize the creation of splashes and/or aerosols.

2. Decontaminate work surfaces after completion of work and after any spill or splash of potentially infectious material with appropriate disinfectant.

3. Decontaminate all cultures, stocks, and other potentially infectious materials before disposal using an effective method. Depending on where the decontamination will be performed, the following methods should be used prior to transport:

    (a) Materials to be decontaminated outside of the immediate laboratory must be placed in a durable, leak proof container and secured for transport.

    (b) Materials to be removed from the facility for decontamination must be packed in accordance with applicable local, state, and federal regulations.

4. A sign incorporating the universal biohazard symbol must be posted at the entrance to the laboratory when infectious agents are present. Posted information must include: the laboratory's biosafety level, the supervisor's name (or other responsible personnel), telephone number, and required procedures for entering and exiting the laboratory. Agent information should be posted in accordance with the institutional policy.

5. An effective integrated pest management program is required.

6. The laboratory supervisor must ensure that laboratory personnel receive appropriate training regarding their duties, the necessary precautions to prevent exposures, and exposure evaluation procedures. Personnel must receive annual updates or additional training when procedural or policy changes occur. Personal health status may impact an individual's susceptibility to infection, ability to receive immunizations or prophylactic interventions. Therefore, all laboratory personnel and particularly women of child-bearing age should be provided with information regarding immune competence and conditions that may predispose them to infection. Individuals having these conditions should be encouraged to self-identify to the institution's healthcare provider for appropriate counseling and guidance.

B. Special Practices

1. All persons entering the laboratory must be advised of the potential hazards and meet specific entry/exit requirements.

2. Laboratory personnel must be provided medical surveillance and offered appropriate immunizations for agents handled or potentially present in the laboratory.

3. Each institution must establish policies and procedures describing the collection and storage of serum samples from at-risk personnel.

4. A laboratory-specific biosafety manual must be prepared and adopted as policy. The biosafety manual must be available and accessible.

5. The laboratory supervisor must ensure that laboratory personnel demonstrate proficiency in standard and special microbiological practices before working with BSL-2 agents.

6. Potentially infectious materials must be placed in a durable, leak proof container during collection, handling, processing, storage, or transport within a facility.

7. Laboratory equipment should be routinely decontaminated, as well as, after spills, splashes, or other potential contamination.

    (a) Spills involving infectious materials must be contained, decontaminated, and cleaned up by staff properly trained and equipped to work with infectious material.

    (b) Equipment must be decontaminated before repair, maintenance, or removal from the laboratory.

8. Incidents that may result in exposure to infectious materials must be immediately evaluated and treated according to procedures described in the laboratory biosafety safety manual. All such incidents must be reported to the laboratory supervisor. Medical evaluation, surveillance, and treatment should be provided and appropriate records maintained.

9. Animals and plants not associated with the work being performed must not be permitted in the laboratory.

10. All procedures involving the manipulation of infectious materials that may generate an aerosol should be conducted within a BSC or other physical containment devices.

C. Safety Equipment (Primary Barriers and Personal Protective Equipment)

1. Properly maintained BSCs (preferably Class II), other appropriate personal protective equipment, or other physical containment devices must be used whenever:

    (a) Procedures with a potential for creating infectious aerosols or splashes are conducted. These may include pipetting, centrifuging, grinding, blending, shaking, mixing, sonicating, opening containers of infectious materials, inoculating animals intranasally, and harvesting infected tissues from animals or eggs.

    (b) High concentrations or large volumes of infectious agents are used. Such materials may be centrifuged in the open laboratory using sealed rotor heads or centrifuge safety cups.

2. Protective laboratory coats, gowns, smocks, or uniforms designated for laboratory use must be worn while working with hazardous materials. Remove protective clothing before leaving for non-laboratory areas (e.g., cafeteria, library, administrative offices). Dispose off protective clothing appropriately, or deposit it for laundering by the institution. It is recommended that laboratory clothing not be taken home.

3. Eye and face protection (goggles, mask, face shield or other splatter guard) is used for anticipated splashes or sprays of infectious or other hazardous materials when the microorganisms must be handled outside the BSC or containment device. Eye and face protection must be disposed off with other contaminated laboratory waste or decontaminated before reuse. Persons who wear contact lenses in laboratories should also wear eye protection.

4. Gloves must be worn to protect hands from exposure to hazardous materials. Glove selection should be based on an appropriate risk assessment. Alternatives to latex gloves should be available. Gloves must not be worn outside the laboratory. In addition, BSL-2 laboratory workers should:

   (a) Change gloves when contaminated, integrity has been compromised, or when otherwise necessary. Wear two pairs of gloves when appropriate.

   (b) Remove gloves and wash hands when work with hazardous materials has been completed and before leaving the laboratory.

   (c) Do not wash or reuse disposable gloves. Dispose off used gloves with other contaminated laboratory waste. Hand washing protocols must be rigorously followed.

5. Eye, face and respiratory protection should be used in rooms containing infected animals as determined by the risk assessment.

D. Laboratory Facilities (Secondary Barriers)

1. Laboratory doors should be self-closing and have locks in accordance with the institutional policies.

2. Laboratories must have a sink for hand washing. The sink may be manually, hands-free, or automatically operated. It should be located near the exit door.

3. The laboratory should be designed so that it can be easily cleaned and decontaminated. Carpets and rugs in laboratories are not permitted.

4. Laboratory furniture must be capable of supporting anticipated loads and uses. Spaces between benches, cabinets, and equipment should be accessible for cleaning.

   (a) Bench tops must be impervious to water and resistant to heat, organic solvents, acids, alkalis, and other chemicals.

    (b) Chairs used in laboratory work must be covered with a non-porous material that can be easily cleaned and decontaminated with appropriate disinfectant.

5. Laboratory windows that open to the exterior are not recommended. However, if a laboratory does have windows that open to the exterior, they must be fitted with screens.

6. BSCs must be installed so that fluctuations of the room air supply and exhaust do not interfere with proper operations. BSCs should be located away from doors, windows that can be opened, heavily traveled laboratory areas, and other possible airflow disruptions.

7. Vacuum lines should be protected with High Efficiency Particulate Air (HEPA) filters, or their equivalent. Filters must be replaced as needed. Liquid disinfectant traps may be required.

8. An eyewash station must be readily available.

9. There are no specific requirements on ventilation systems. However, planning of new facilities should consider mechanical ventilation systems that provide an inward flow of air without recirculation to spaces outside of the laboratory.

10. HEPA filtered exhaust air from a Class II BSC can be safely re-circulated back into the laboratory environment if the cabinet is tested and certified at least annually and operated according to manufacturer's recommendations. BSCs can also be connected to the laboratory exhaust system by either a thimble (canopy) connection or a direct (hard) connection. Provisions to assure proper safety cabinet performance and air system operation must be verified.

11. A method for decontaminating all laboratory wastes should be available in the facility (e.g., autoclave, chemical disinfection, incineration, or other validated decontamination method).

Biosafety Level 3

It is applicable to clinical, diagnostic, teaching, research, or production facilities where work is performed with indigenous or exotic agents that may cause serious or potentially lethal disease through inhalation route exposure. Laboratory personnel must receive specific training in handling pathogenic and potentially lethal agents, and must be supervised by scientists competent in handling infectious agents and associated procedures.

All procedures involving the manipulation of infectious materials must be conducted within BSCs, other physical containment devices, or by personnel wearing appropriate personal protective equipment.

A BSL-3 laboratory has special engineering and design features.

The following standard and special safety practices, equipment, and facility requirements apply to BSL-3:

A. Standard Microbiological Practices

1. The laboratory supervisor must enforce the institutional policies that control access to the laboratory.

2. Persons must wash their hands after working with potentially hazardous materials and before leaving the laboratory.

3. Eating, drinking, smoking, handling contact lenses, applying cosmetics, and storing food for human consumption must not be permitted in laboratory areas. Food must be stored outside the laboratory area in cabinets or refrigerators designated and used for this purpose.

4. Mouth pipetting is prohibited; mechanical pipetting devices must be used.

5. Policies for the safe handling of sharps, such as needles, scalpels, pipettes, and broken glassware must be developed and implemented. Whenever practical, laboratory supervisors should adopt improved engineering and work practice controls that reduce risk of sharps injuries.

Precautions, including those listed below, must always be taken with sharp items. These include:

(a) Careful management of needles and other sharps are of primary importance. Needles must not be bent, sheared, broken, recapped, removed from disposable syringes, or otherwise manipulated by hand before disposal.

(b) Used disposable needles and syringes must be carefully placed in conveniently located puncture-resistant containers used for sharps disposal.

(c) Non-disposable sharps must be placed in a hard walled container for transport to a processing area for decontamination, preferably by autoclaving.

(d) Broken glassware must not be handled directly. Instead, it must be removed using a brush and dustpan, tongs, or forceps. Plasticware should be substituted for glassware whenever possible.

1. Perform all procedures to minimize the creation of splashes and/or aerosols.

2. Decontaminate work surfaces after completion of work and after any spill or splash of potentially infectious material with appropriate disinfectant.

3. Decontaminate all cultures, stocks, and other potentially infectious materials before disposal using an effective method. A method for decontaminating all laboratory wastes should be available in the facility, preferably within the laboratory (e.g., autoclave, chemical disinfection, incineration, or other validated decontamination method). Depending on where the decontamination will be performed, the following methods should be used prior to transport:

   (a) Materials to be decontaminated outside of the immediate laboratory must be placed in a durable, leak proof container and secured for transport.

   (b) Materials to be removed from the facility for decontamination must be packed in accordance with applicable local, state, and federal regulations.

4. A sign incorporating the universal biohazard symbol must be posted at the entrance to the laboratory when infectious agents are present. Posted information must include the laboratory's biosafety level, the supervisor's name (or other responsible personnel), telephone number, and required procedures for entering and exiting the laboratory. Agent information should be posted in accordance with the institutional policy.

5. An effective integrated pest management program is required.

6. The laboratory supervisor must ensure that laboratory personnel receive appropriate training regarding their duties, the necessary precautions to prevent exposures, and exposure evaluation procedures. Personnel must receive annual updates or additional training when procedural or policy changes occur. Personal health status may impact an individual's susceptibility to infection, ability to receive immunizations or prophylactic interventions. Therefore, all laboratory personnel and particularly women of child-bearing age should be provided with information regarding immune competence and conditions that may predispose them to infection. Individuals having these conditions should be encouraged to self-identify to the institution's healthcare provider for appropriate counseling and guidance.

B. Special Practices

1. All persons entering the laboratory must be advised of the potential hazards and meet specific entry/exit requirements.

2. Laboratory personnel must be provided medical surveillance and offered appropriate immunizations for agents handled or potentially present in the laboratory.

3. Each institution must establish policies and procedures describing the collection and storage of serum samples from at-risk personnel.

4. A laboratory-specific biosafety manual must be prepared and adopted as policy. The biosafety manual must be available and accessible.

5. The laboratory supervisor must ensure that laboratory personnel demonstrate proficiency in standard and special microbiological practices before working with BSL-3 agents.

6. Potentially infectious materials must be placed in a durable, leak proof container during collection, handling, processing, storage, or transport within a facility.

7. Laboratory equipment should be routinely decontaminated, as well as, after spills, splashes, or other potential contamination.

    (a) Spills involving infectious materials must be contained, decontaminated, and cleaned up by staff properly trained and equipped to work with infectious material.

    (b) Equipment must be decontaminated before repair, maintenance, or removal from the laboratory.

8. Incidents that may result in exposure to infectious materials must be immediately evaluated and treated according to procedures described in the laboratory biosafety safety manual. All such incidents must be reported to the laboratory supervisor. Medical evaluation, surveillance, and treatment should be provided and appropriate records maintained.

9. Animals and plants not associated with the work being performed must not be permitted in the laboratory.

10. All procedures involving the manipulation of infectious materials must be conducted within a BSC, or other physical containment devices. No work with open vessels is conducted on the bench. When a procedure cannot be performed within a BSC, a combination of personal protective equipment and other containment devices, such as a centrifuge safety cup or sealed rotor, must be used.

C. Safety Equipment (Primary Barriers and Personal Protective Equipment)

1. All procedures involving the manipulation of infectious materials must be conducted within a BSC (preferably Class II or Class III), or other physical containment devices.

2. Protective laboratory clothing with a solid-front such as tie-back or wraparound gowns, scrub suits, or coveralls are worn by workers when in the laboratory. Protective clothing is not worn outside of the laboratory. Reusable clothing is decontaminated with appropriate disinfectant before being laundered. Clothing is changed when contaminated.

3. Eye and face protection (goggles, mask, face shield or other splatter guard) is used for anticipated splashes or sprays of infectious or other hazardous materials. Eye and face protection must be disposed of with other contaminated laboratory waste or decontaminated before reuse. Persons who wear contact lenses in laboratories must also wear eye protection.

4. Gloves must be worn to protect hands from exposure to hazardous materials. Glove selection should be based on an appropriate risk assessment. Alternatives to latex gloves should be available. Gloves must not be worn outside the laboratory. In addition, BSL-3 laboratory workers should:

    (a) Change gloves when contaminated, integrity has been compromised, or when otherwise necessary. Wear two pairs of gloves when appropriate.

    (b) Remove gloves and wash hands when work with hazardous materials has been completed and before leaving the laboratory.

    (c) Do not wash or reuse disposable gloves. Dispose of used gloves with other contaminated laboratory waste. Hand washing protocols must be rigorously followed.

5. Eye, face, and respiratory protection must be used in rooms containing infected animals.

D. Laboratory Facilities (Secondary Barriers)

1. Laboratory doors must be self closing and have locks in accordance with the institutional policies. The laboratory must be separated from areas that are open to unrestricted traffic flow within the building. Access to the laboratory is restricted to entry by a series of two self-closing doors. A clothing change

room (anteroom) may be included in the passageway between the two self-closing doors.

2. Laboratories must have a sink for hand washing. The sink must be hands-free or automatically operated. It should be located near the exit door. If the laboratory is segregated into different laboratories, a sink must also be available for hand washing in each zone. Additional sinks may be required as determined by the risk assessment.

3. The laboratory must be designed so that it can be easily cleaned and decontaminated. Carpets and rugs are not permitted. Seams, floors, walls, and ceiling surfaces should be sealed. Spaces around doors and ventilation openings should be capable of being sealed to facilitate space decontamination.

    (a) Floors must be slip resistant, impervious to liquids, and resistant to chemicals. Consideration should be given to the installation of seamless, sealed, resilient or poured floors, with integral cove bases.

    (b) Walls should be constructed to produce a sealed smooth finish that can be easily cleaned and decontaminated.

    (c) Ceilings should be constructed, sealed, and finished in the same general manner as walls. Decontamination of the entire laboratory should be considered when there has been gross contamination of the space, significant changes in laboratory usage, for major renovations, or maintenance shut downs. Selection of the appropriate materials and methods used to decontaminate the laboratory must be based on the risk assessment of the biological agents in use.

4. Laboratory furniture must be capable of supporting anticipated loads and uses. Spaces between benches, cabinets, and equipment must be accessible for cleaning.

    (a) Bench tops must be impervious to water and resistant to heat, organic solvents, acids, alkalis, and other chemicals.

    (b) Chairs used in laboratory work must be covered with a non-porous material that can be easily cleaned and decontaminated with appropriate disinfectant.

5. All windows in the laboratory must be sealed.

6. BSCs must be installed so that fluctuations of the room air supply and exhaust do not interfere with proper operations. BSCs should be located away from doors, heavily traveled laboratory areas, and other possible airflow disruptions.

7. Vacuum lines must be protected with HEPA filters, or their equivalent. Filters must be replaced as needed. Liquid disinfectant traps may be required.

8. An eyewash station must be readily available in the laboratory.

9. A ducted air ventilation system is required. This system must provide sustained directional airflow by drawing air into the laboratory from "clean" areas toward "potentially contaminated" areas. The laboratory shall be designed such that under failure conditions the airflow will not be reversed.

    (a) Laboratory personnel must be able to verify directional air flow. A visual monitoring device which confirms directional air flow must be provided at the laboratory entry. Audible alarms should be considered to notify personnel of air flow disruption.

    (b) The laboratory exhaust air must not re-circulate to any other area of the building.

    (c) The laboratory building exhaust air should be dispersed away from occupied areas and from building air intake locations or the exhaust air must be HEPA filtered.

10. HEPA filtered exhaust air from a Class II BSC can be safely re-circulated into the laboratory environment if the cabinet is tested and certified at least annually and operated according to manufacturer's recommendations. BSCs can also be connected to the laboratory exhaust system by either a thimble (canopy) connection or a direct (hard) connection. Provisions to assure proper safety cabinet performance and air system operation must be verified. BSCs should be certified at least annually to assure correct performance. Class III BSCs must be directly (hard) connected up through the second exhaust HEPA filter of the cabinet. Supply air must be provided in such a manner that prevents positive pressurization of the cabinet.

11. A method for decontaminating all laboratory wastes should be available in the facility, preferably within the laboratory (e.g., autoclave, chemical disinfection, incineration, or other validated decontamination method).

12. Equipment that may produce infectious aerosols must be contained in devices that exhaust air through HEPA filtration or other equivalent technology before being discharged into the laboratory. These HEPA filters should be tested and/or replaced at least annually.

13. Facility design consideration should be given to means of decontaminating large pieces of equipment before removal from the laboratory.

14. Enhanced environmental and personal protection may be required by the agent summary statement, risk assessment, or applicable local, state, or federal regulations. These laboratory enhancements may include, for example, one or more of the following; an anteroom for clean storage of equipment and supplies with dress-in, shower-out capabilities; gas tight dampers to facilitate laboratory isolation; final HEPA filtration of the laboratory exhaust air; laboratory effluent decontamination; and advanced access control devices such as biometrics. HEPA filter housings should have gas-tight isolation dampers; decontamination ports; and/or bag-in/bag-out (with appropriate decontamination procedures) capability. The HEPA filter housing should allow for leak testing of each filter and assembly. The filters and the housing should be certified at least annually.

15. The BSL-3 facility design, operational parameters, and procedures must be verified and documented prior to operation. Facilities must be re-verified and documented at least annually.

Biosafety Level 4

It is required for work with dangerous and exotic agents that pose a high individual risk of life-threatening disease, aerosol transmission, or related agent with unknown risk of transmission. Agents with a close or identical antigenic relationship to agents requiring BSL-4 containment must be handled at this level until sufficient data are obtained either to confirm continued work at this level, or re-designate the level. Laboratory staff must have specific and thorough training in handling extremely hazardous infectious agents. Laboratory staff must understand the primary and secondary containment functions of standard and special practices, containment equipment, and laboratory design characteristics. All laboratory staff and supervisors must be competent in handling agents and procedures requiring BSL-4 containment. Access to the laboratory is controlled by the laboratory supervisor in accordance with institutional policies.

There are two models for BSL-4 laboratories:

1. A *Cabinet Laboratory* where all handling of agents must be performed in a Class III BSC.

2. A *Suit Laboratory* where personnel must wear a positive pressure protective suit.

3. BSL-4 Cabinet and Suit Laboratories have special engineering and design features to prevent microorganisms from being disseminated into the environment. The following standard and special safety practices, equipment, and facilities apply to BSL-4:

A. Standard Microbiological Practices

1. The laboratory supervisor must enforce the institutional policies that control access to the laboratory.

2. All persons leaving the laboratory must be required to take a personal body shower.

3. Eating, drinking, smoking, handling contact lenses, applying cosmetics, and storing food for human consumption must not be permitted in laboratory areas. Food must be stored outside the laboratory area in cabinets or refrigerators designated and used for this purpose.

4. Mechanical pipetting devices must be used.

5. Policies for the safe handling of sharps, such as needles, scalpels, pipettes, and broken glassware must be developed and implemented. Precautions, including those listed below, must be taken with any sharp items. These include:

    (a) Broken glassware must not be handled directly. Instead, it must be removed using a brush and dustpan, tongs, or forceps. Plasticware should be substituted for glassware whenever possible.

    (b) Use of needles and syringes or other sharp instruments should be restricted in the laboratory, except when there is no practical alternative.

    (c) Used needles must not be bent, sheared, broken, recapped, removed from disposable syringes, or otherwise manipulated by hand before disposal or decontamination. Used disposable needles must be carefully placed in puncture-resistant containers used for sharps disposal, located as close to the point of use as possible.

    (d) Whenever practical, laboratory supervisors should adopt improved engineering and work practice controls that reduce risk of sharps injuries.

6. Perform all procedures to minimize the creation of splashes and/or aerosols.

7. Decontaminate work surfaces with appropriate disinfectant after completion of work and after any spill or splash of potentially infectious material.

8. Decontaminate all wastes before removal from the laboratory by an effective and validated method.

9. A sign incorporating the universal biohazard symbol must be posted at the entrance to the laboratory when infectious agents are present. Posted information must include the laboratory's biosafety level, the supervisor's name (or other responsible personnel), telephone number, and required procedures for entering and exiting the laboratory. Agent information should be posted in accordance with the institutional policy.

10. An effective integrated pest management program is required.

11. The laboratory supervisor must ensure that laboratory personnel receive appropriate training regarding their duties, the necessary precautions to prevent exposures, and exposure evaluation procedures. Personnel must receive annual updates or additional training when procedural or policy changes occur. Personal health status may impact an individual's susceptibility to infection, ability to receive immunizations or prophylactic interventions. Therefore, all laboratory personnel and particularly women of child-bearing age should be provided with information regarding immune competence and conditions that may predispose them to infection. Individuals having these conditions should be encouraged to self-identify to the institution's healthcare provider for appropriate counseling and guidance.

B. Special Practices

1. All persons entering the laboratory must be advised of the potential hazards and meet specific entry/exit requirements in accordance with institutional policies. Only persons whose presence in the facility or individual laboratory rooms is required for scientific or support purposes should be authorized to enter. Entry into the facility must be limited by means of secure, locked doors. A logbook, or other means of documenting the date and time of all persons entering and leaving the laboratory must be maintained. While the laboratory is operational, personnel must enter and exit the laboratory through the clothing change and shower rooms

except during emergencies. All personal clothing must be removed in the outer clothing change room. Laboratory clothing, including undergarments, pants, shirts, jumpsuits, shoes, and gloves, must be used by all personnel entering the laboratory. All persons leaving the laboratory must take a personal body shower. Used laboratory clothing must not be removed from the inner change room through the personal shower. These items must be treated as contaminated materials and decontaminated before laundering. After the laboratory has been completely decontaminated, necessary staff may enter and exit without following the clothing change and shower requirements described above.

2. Laboratory personnel and support staff must be provided appropriate occupational medical service including medical surveillance and available immunizations for agents handled or potentially present in the laboratory. A system must be established for reporting and documenting laboratory accidents, exposures, employee absenteeism and for the medical surveillance of potential laboratory-associated illnesses. An essential adjunct to such an occupational medical services system is the availability of a facility for the isolation and medical care of personnel with potential or known laboratory acquired infections.

3. Each institution must establish policies and procedures describing the collection and storage of serum samples from at-risk personnel.

4. A laboratory-specific biosafety manual must be prepared. The Biosafety manual must be available, accessible, and followed.

5. The laboratory supervisor is responsible for ensuring that laboratory personnel:

    (a) Demonstrate high proficiency in standard and special microbiological practices, and techniques for working with agents requiring BSL-4 containment.

    (b) Receive appropriate training in the practices and operations specific to the laboratory facility.

    (c) Receive annual updates or additional training when procedural or policy changes occur.

6. Removal of biological materials that are to remain in a viable or intact state from the laboratory must be transferred to a non-breakable, sealed primary container and then enclosed in a non-breakable, sealed secondary container. These materials

must be transferred through a disinfectant dunk tank, fumigation chamber, or decontamination shower. Once removed, packaged viable material must not be opened outside BSL-4 containment unless inactivated by a validated method.

7. Laboratory equipment must be routinely decontaminated, as well as after spills, splashes, or other potential contamination.

    (a) Spills involving infectious materials must be contained, decontaminated, and cleaned up by appropriate professional staff, or others properly trained and equipped to work with infectious material. A spill procedure must be developed and posted within the laboratory.

    (b) Equipment must be decontaminated using an effective and validated method before repair, maintenance, or removal from the laboratory. The interior of the Class III cabinet as well as all contaminated plenums, fans and filters must be decontaminated using a validated gaseous or vapor method.

    (c) Equipment or material that might be damaged by high temperatures or steam must be decontaminated using an effective and validated procedure such as a gaseous or vapor method in an airlock or chamber designed for this purpose.

8. Incidents that may result in exposure to infectious materials must be immediately evaluated and treated according to procedures described in the laboratory biosafety manual. All incidents must be reported to the laboratory supervisor, institutional management and appropriate laboratory personnel as defined in the laboratory biosafety manual. Medical evaluation, surveillance, and treatment should be provided and appropriate records maintained.

9. Animals and plants not associated with the work being performed must not be permitted in the laboratory.

10. Supplies and materials that are not brought into the BSL-4 laboratory through the change room must be brought in through a previously decontaminated double-door autoclave, fumigation chamber, or airlock. After securing the outer doors, personnel within the laboratory retrieve the materials by opening the interior doors of the autoclave, fumigation chamber, or airlock. These doors must be secured after materials are brought into the facility. The doors of the

autoclave are interlocked in a manner that prevents opening of the outer door unless the autoclave has been operated through a decontamination cycle. The doors of a fumigation chamber must be secured in a manner that prevents opening of the outer door unless the fumigation chamber has been operated through a fumigation cycle. Only necessary equipment and supplies should be stored inside the BSL-4 laboratory. All equipment and supplies taken inside the laboratory must be decontaminated before removal from the facility.

11. Daily inspections of essential containment and life support systems must be completed and documented before laboratory work is initiated to ensure that the laboratory is operating according to established parameters.

12. Practical and effective protocols for emergency situations must be established. These protocols must include plans for medical emergencies, facility malfunctions, fires, escape of animals within the laboratory, and other potential emergencies. Training in emergency response procedures must be provided to emergency response personnel and other responsible staff according to institutional policies.

C. Safety Equipment (Primary Barriers and Personal Protective Equipment)

Cabinet Laboratory

1. All manipulations of infectious materials within the facility must be conducted in the Class III biological safety cabinet. Double-door, pass through autoclaves must be provided for decontaminating materials passing out of the Class III BSC(s). The autoclave doors must be interlocked so that only one can be opened at any time and be automatically controlled so that the outside door to the autoclave can only be opened after the decontamination cycle has been completed. The Class III cabinet must also have a pass-through dunk tank, fumigation chamber, or equivalent decontamination method so that materials and equipment that cannot be decontaminated in the autoclave can be safely removed from the cabinet. Containment must be maintained at all times. The Class III cabinet must have a HEPA filter on the supply air intake and two HEPA filters in series on the exhaust outlet of the unit. There must be gas tight dampers on the supply and exhaust ducts of the cabinet to permit gas or vapor decontamination of the unit. Ports for injection of test medium must be present on all HEPA filter

housings. The interior of the Class III cabinet must be constructed with smooth finishes that can be easily cleaned and decontaminated. All sharp edges on cabinet finishes must be eliminated to reduce the potential for cuts and tears of gloves. Equipment to be placed in the Class III cabinet should also be free of sharp edges or other surfaces that may damage or puncture the cabinet gloves. Class III cabinet gloves must be inspected for leaks periodically and changed if necessary. Gloves should be replaced annually during cabinet recertification. The cabinet should be designed to permit maintenance and repairs of cabinet mechanical systems (refrigeration, incubators, centrifuges, etc.) to be performed from the exterior of the cabinet whenever possible. Manipulation of high concentrations or large volumes of infectious agents within the Class III cabinet should be performed using physical containment devices inside the cabinet whenever practical. Such materials should be centrifuged inside the cabinet using sealed rotor heads or centrifuge safety cups. The Class III cabinet must be certified at least annually.

2. Protective laboratory clothing with a solid-front such as tie-back or wrap around gowns, scrub suits, or coveralls must be worn by workers when in the laboratory. No personal clothing, jewelry, or other items except eyeglasses should be taken past the personal shower area. All protective clothing must be removed in the dirty side change room before showering. Reusable clothing must be autoclaved before being laundered.

3. Eye, face and respiratory protection should be used in rooms containing infected animals as determined by the risk assessment. Prescription eyeglasses must be decontaminated before removal through the personal body shower.

4. Gloves must be worn to protect against breaks or tears in the cabinet gloves. Gloves must not be worn outside the laboratory. Alternatives to latex gloves should be available. Do not wash or reuse disposable gloves. Dispose of used gloves with other contaminated laboratory waste.

Suit Laboratory

1. All procedures must be conducted by personnel wearing a one-piece positive pressure suit ventilated with a life support system. All manipulations of infectious agents must be performed within a BSC or other primary barrier system.

Equipment that may produce aerosols must be contained in devices that exhaust air through HEPA filtration before being discharged into the laboratory. These HEPA filters should be tested annually and replaced as needed. HEPA filtered exhaust air from a Class II BSC can be safely re-circulated into the laboratory environment if the cabinet is tested and certified at least annually and operated according to manufacturer's recommendations.

2. Protective laboratory clothing such as scrub suits must be worn by workers before entering the room used for donning positive pressure suits. All protective clothing must be removed in the dirty side change room before entering the personal shower. Reusable laboratory clothing must be autoclaved before being laundered.

3. Inner gloves must be worn to protect against break or tears in the outer suit gloves. Disposable gloves must not be worn outside the change area. Alternatives to latex gloves should be available. Do not wash or reuse disposable gloves. Inner gloves must be removed and discarded in the inner change room prior to personal shower. Dispose of used gloves with other contaminated waste.

4. Decontamination of outer suit gloves is performed during operations to remove gross contamination and minimize further contamination of the laboratory.

D. Laboratory Facilities (Secondary Barriers)

Cabinet Laboratory

1. The BSL-4 cabinet laboratory consists of either a separate building or a clearly demarcated and isolated zone within a building. Laboratory doors must have locks in accordance with the institutional policies. Rooms in the facility must be arranged to ensure sequential passage through an inner (dirty) changing area, a personal shower and an outer (clean) change room prior to exiting the room(s) containing the Class III BSC(s). An automatically activated emergency power source must be provided at a minimum for the laboratory exhaust system, life support systems, alarms, lighting, entry and exit controls, BSCs, and door gaskets. Monitoring and control systems for air supply, exhaust, life support, alarms, entry and exit, and security systems should be on an uninterrupted power supply (UPS). A double-door autoclave, dunk tank, fumigation chamber, or ventilated anteroom/airlock must be

provided at the containment barrier for the passage of materials, supplies, or equipment.

2. A hands-free sink must be provided near the door of the cabinet room(s) and the inner change room. A sink must be provided in the outer change room. All sinks in the room(s) containing the Class III BSC and the inner (dirty) change room must be connected to the wastewater decontamination system.

3. Walls, floors, and ceilings of the laboratory must be constructed to form a sealed internal shell to facilitate fumigation and prohibit animal and insect intrusion. The internal surfaces of this shell must be resistant to liquids and chemicals used for cleaning and decontamination of the area. Floors must be monolithic, sealed and coved. All penetrations in the internal shell of the laboratory and inner change room must be sealed. Openings around doors into the cabinet room and inner change room must be minimized and capable of being sealed to facilitate decontamination. Drains in the laboratory floor (if present) must be connected directly to the liquid waste decontamination system. Services, plumbing or otherwise that penetrate the laboratory walls, floors, ceiling, plumbing or otherwise, must ensure that no backflow from the laboratory occurs. These penetrations must be fitted with two (in series) backflow prevention devices. Consideration should be given to locating these devices outside of containment. Atmospheric venting systems must be provided with two HEPA filters in series and be sealed up to the second filter. Decontamination of the entire cabinet must be performed using a validated gaseous or vapor method when there have been significant changes in cabinet usage, before major renovations or maintenance shut downs, and in other situations, as determined by risk assessment. Selection of the appropriate materials and methods used for decontamination must be based on the risk assessment of the biological agents in use.

4. Laboratory furniture must be of simple construction, capable of supporting anticipated loading and uses. Spaces between benches, cabinets, and equipment must be accessible for cleaning and decontamination. Chairs and other furniture should be covered with a non-porous material that can be easily decontaminated.

5. Windows must be break-resistant and sealed.

6. If Class II BSCs are needed in the cabinet laboratory, they must be installed so that fluctuations of the room air supply and

exhaust do not interfere with proper operations. Class II cabinets should be located away from doors, heavily traveled laboratory areas, and other possible airflow disruptions.

7. Central vacuum systems are not recommended. If, however, there is a central vacuum system, it must not serve areas outside the cabinet room. Two in-line HEPA filters must be placed near each use point. Filters must be installed to permit in-place decontamination and replacement.

8. An eyewash station must be readily available in the laboratory.

9. A dedicated non-recirculation ventilation system is provided. Only laboratories with the same HVAC requirements (i.e., other BSL-4 labs, ABSL-4, BSL-3 Ag labs) may share ventilation systems if each individual laboratory system is isolated by gas tight dampers and HEPA filters. The supply and exhaust components of the ventilation system must be designed to maintain the laboratory at negative pressure to surrounding areas and provide differential pressure/directional airflow between adjacent areas within the laboratory. Redundant supply fans are recommended. Redundant exhaust fans are required. Supply and exhaust fans must be interlocked to prevent positive pressurization of the laboratory. The ventilation system must be monitored and alarmed to indicate malfunction or deviation from design parameters. A visual monitoring device must be installed near the clean change room so proper differential pressures within the laboratory may be verified. Supply air to and exhaust air from the cabinet room, inner change room, and fumigation/decontamination chambers must pass through HEPA filter(s). The air exhaust discharge must be located away from occupied spaces and building air intakes. All HEPA filters should be located as near as practicable to the cabinet or laboratory in order to minimize the length of potentially contaminated ductwork. All HEPA filters must to be tested and certified annually. The HEPA filter housings should be designed to allow for *in situ* decontamination and validation of the filter prior to removal. The design of the HEPA filter housing must have gas-tight isolation dampers; decontamination ports; and ability to scan each filter assembly for leaks.

10. HEPA filtered exhaust air from a Class II BSC can be safely re-circulated into the laboratory environment if the cabinet is tested and certified at least annually and operated according to the manufacturer's recommendations. BSCs can also be

connected to the laboratory exhaust system by either a thimble (canopy) connection or a direct (hard) connection. Provisions to assure proper safety cabinet performance and air system operation must be verified. Class III BSCs must be directly and independently exhausted through two HEPA filters in series. Supply air must be provided in such a manner that prevents positive pressurization of the cabinet.

11. Pass through dunk tanks, fumigation chambers, or equivalent decontamination methods must be provided so that materials and equipment that cannot be decontaminated in the autoclave can be safely removed from the cabinet room(s). Access to the exit side of the pass-through shall be limited to those individuals authorized to be in the BSL-4 laboratory.

12. Liquid effluents from cabinet room sinks, floor drains, autoclave chambers, and other sources within the cabinet room must be decontaminated by a proven method, preferably heat treatment, before being discharged to the sanitary sewer. Decontamination of all liquid wastes must be documented. The decontamination process for liquid wastes must be validated physically and biologically. Biological validation must be performed annually or more often if required by institutional policy. Effluents from showers and toilets may be discharged to the sanitary sewer without treatment.

13. A double-door, pass through autoclave(s) must be provided for decontaminating materials passing out of the cabinet laboratory. Autoclaves that open outside of the laboratory must be sealed to the primary wall. This bioseal must be durable and airtight. Positioning the bioseal so that the equipment can be accessed and maintained from outside the laboratory is strongly recommended. The autoclave doors must be interlocked so that only one can be opened at any time and be automatically controlled so that the outside door to the autoclave can only be opened after the decontamination cycle has been completed. Gas and liquid discharge from the autoclave chamber must be decontaminated. When feasible, autoclave decontamination processes should be designed so that over-pressurization cannot release unfiltered air or steam exposed to infectious material to the environment.

14. The BSL-4 facility design parameters and operational procedures must be documented. The facility must be tested to verify that the design and operational parameters have been met prior to operation. Facilities must also be re-verified

annually. Verification criteria should be modified as necessary by operational experience.

15. Appropriate communication systems must be provided between the laboratory and the outside (e.g., voice, fax, and computer). Provisions for emergency communication and access/egress must be considered.

Suit Laboratory

1. The BSL-4 suit laboratory consists of either a separate building or a clearly demarcated and isolated zone within a building. Laboratory doors must have locks in accordance with the institutional policies. Rooms in the facility must be arranged to ensure exit by sequential passage through the chemical shower, inner (dirty) change room, personal shower, and outer (clean) changing area. Entry into the BSL-4 laboratory must be through an airlock fitted with airtight doors. Personnel who enter this area must wear a positive pressure suit with HEPA filtered breathing air. The breathing air systems must have redundant compressors, failure alarms and emergency backup. A chemical shower must be provided to decontaminate the surface of the positive pressure suit before the worker leaves the laboratory. In the event of an emergency exit or failure of chemical shower system a method for decontaminating positive pressure suits, such as a gravity fed supply of chemical disinfectant, is needed. An automatically activated emergency power source must be provided at a minimum for the laboratory exhaust system, life support systems, alarms, lighting, entry and exit controls, BSCs, and door gaskets. Monitoring and control systems for air supply, exhaust, life support, alarms, entry and exit, and security systems should be on a UPS. A double-door autoclave, dunk tank, or fumigation chamber must be provided at the containment barrier for the passage of materials, supplies, or equipment.

2. Sinks inside the suit laboratory should be placed near procedure areas and contain traps and be connected to the wastewater decontamination system.

3. Walls, floors, and ceilings of the laboratory must be constructed to form a sealed internal shell to facilitate fumigation and prohibit animal and insect intrusion. The internal surfaces of this shell must be resistant to liquids and chemicals used for cleaning and decontamination of the area. Floors must be monolithic, sealed and coved. All penetrations in the internal shell of the laboratory, suit storage room and the inner change

room must be sealed. Drains if present, in the laboratory floor must be connected directly to the liquid waste decontamination system. Sewer vents and other service lines must be protected by two HEPA filters in series and have protection against insect and animal intrusion. Services, plumbing or otherwise that penetrate the laboratory walls, floors, ceiling, plumbing or otherwise, must ensure that no backflow from the laboratory occurs. These penetrations must be fitted with two (in series) backflow prevention devices. Consideration should be given to locating these devices outside of containment. Atmospheric venting systems must be provided with two HEPA filters in series and be sealed up to the second filter. Decontamination of the entire laboratory must be performed using a validated gaseous or vapor method when there have been significant changes in laboratory usage, before major renovations or maintenance shut downs, and in other situations, as determined by risk assessment.

4. Laboratory furniture must be of simple construction, capable of supporting anticipated loading and uses. Sharp edges and corners should be avoided. Spaces between benches, cabinets, and equipment must be accessible for cleaning and decontamination. Chairs and other furniture should be covered with a non-porous material that can be easily decontaminated.

5. Windows must be break-resistant and sealed.

6. BSCs and other primary containment barrier systems must be installed so that fluctuations of the room air supply and exhaust do not interfere with proper operations. BSCs should be located away from doors, heavily traveled laboratory areas, and other possible airflow disruptions.

7. Central vacuum systems are not recommended. If, however, there is a central vacuum system, it must not serve areas outside the BSL-4 laboratory. Two inline HEPA filters must be placed near each use point. Filters must be installed to permit in-place decontamination and replacement.

8. An eyewash station must be readily available in the laboratory area for use during maintenance and repair activities.

9. A dedicated non-recirculating ventilation system is provided. Only laboratories with the same HVAC requirements (i.e., other BSL-4 labs, ABSL-4, BSL-3 Ag labs) may share ventilation systems if each individual laboratory system is isolated by gas tight dampers and HEPA filters. The supply and exhaust

components of the ventilation system must be designed to maintain the laboratory at negative pressure to surrounding areas and provide differential pressure/directional airflow between adjacent areas within the laboratory. Redundant supply fans are recommended. Redundant exhaust fans are required. Supply and exhaust fans must be interlocked to prevent positive pressurization of the laboratory. The ventilation system must be monitored and alarmed to indicate malfunction or deviation from design parameters. A visual monitoring device must be installed near the clean change room so proper differential pressures within the laboratory may be verified. Supply air to the laboratory, including the decontamination shower, must pass through a HEPA filter. All exhaust air from the suit laboratory, decontamination shower and fumigation or decontamination chambers must pass through two HEPA filters, in series, before discharge to the outside. The exhaust air discharge must be located away from occupied spaces and air intakes. All HEPA filters must be located as near as practicable to the laboratory in order to minimize the length of potentially contaminated ductwork. All HEPA filters must be tested and certified annually. The HEPA filter housings should be designed to allow for *in situ* decontamination and validation of the filter prior to removal. The design of the HEPA filter housing must have gas-tight isolation dampers; decontamination ports; and ability to scan each filter assembly for leaks.

10. HEPA filtered exhaust air from a Class II BSC can be safely re-circulated back into the laboratory environment if the cabinet is tested and certified at least annually and operated according to the manufacturer's recommendations. Biological safety cabinets can also be connected to the laboratory exhaust system by either a thimble (canopy) connection or a direct (hard) connection. Provisions to assure proper safety cabinet performance and air system operation must be verified.

11. Pass through dunk tanks, fumigation chambers, or equivalent decontamination methods must be provided so that materials and equipment that cannot be decontaminated in the autoclave can be safely removed from the BSL-4 laboratory. Access to the exit side of the pass-through shall be limited to those individuals authorized to be in the BSL-4 laboratory.

12. Liquid effluents from chemical showers, sinks, floor drains, autoclave chambers, and other sources within the laboratory

must be decontaminated by a proven method, preferably heat treatment, before being discharged to the sanitary sewer. Decontamination of all liquid wastes must be documented. The decontamination process for liquid wastes must be validated physically and biologically. Biological validation must be performed annually or more often if required by institutional policy. Effluents from personal body showers and toilets may be discharged to the sanitary sewer without treatment.

13. A double-door, pass through autoclave(s) must be provided for decontaminating materials passing out of the cabinet laboratory. Autoclaves that open outside of the laboratory must be sealed to the primary wall. This bioseal must be durable and airtight. Positioning the bioseal so that the equipment can be accessed and maintained from outside the laboratory is strongly recommended. The autoclave doors must be interlocked so that only one can be opened at any time and be automatically controlled so that the outside door to the autoclave can only be opened after the decontamination cycle has been completed. Gas and liquid discharge from the autoclave chamber must be decontaminated. When feasible, autoclave decontamination processes should be designed so that over-pressurization cannot release unfiltered air or steam exposed to infectious material to the environment.

14. The BSL-4 facility design parameters and operational procedures must be documented. The facility must be tested to verify that the design and operational parameters have been met prior to operation. Facilities must also be re-verified annually. Verification criteria should be modified as necessary by operational experience.

15. Appropriate communication systems must be provided between the laboratory and the outside (e.g., voice, fax, and computer). Provisions for emergency communication and access/egress should be considered.

Biosafety Level on Indian Perspective

The Government of India had proposed safety levels for work with recombinant DNA technique take into consideration the source of the donor DNA and its disease-producing potential. These four levels corresponds to (P1<P2<P3<P4) facilities approximate to 4 risk groups assigned for etiologic agents.

These levels and the appropriate conditions are enumerated as follows:

Biosafety Level 1 (P1): These practices, safety equipment and facilities are appropriate for undergraduate and secondary educational training and teaching laboratories and for other facilities in which work is done with defined and characterized strains of viable microorganisms not known to cause disease in healthy adult human. No special accommodation or equipment is required but the laboratory personnel are required to have specific training and to be supervised by a scientist with general training in microbiology or a related science.

Biosafety Level 2 (P2): These practices, safety equipment and facilities are applicable in clinical, diagnostic, teaching and other facilities in which work is done with the broad spectrum of indigenous moderate-risk agents present in the community and associated with human disease of varying severity. Laboratory workers are required to have specific training in handling pathogenic agents and to be supervised by competent scientists. Accommodation and facilities including safety cabinets are prescribed, especially for handling large volume are high concentrations of agents when aerosols are likely to be created. Access to the laboratory is controlled.

Biosafety level 3 (P3): These practices, safety equipment and facilities are applicable to clinical, diagnostic, teaching research or production facilities in which work is done with indigenous or exotic agents where the potential for infection by aerosols is real and the disease may have serious or lethal consequences. Personnel are required to have specific training in work with these agents and to be supervised by scientists experienced in this kind of microbiology. Specially designed laboratories and precautions including the use of safety cabinets are prescribed and the access is strictly controlled.

Biosafety level 4 (P4): These practices, safety equipment and facilities are applicable to work with dangerous and exotic agents which pose a high individual risk of life-threatening disease. Strict training and supervision are required and the work is done in specially designed laboratories under stringent safety conditions, including the use of safety cabinets and positive pressure personnel suits. Access is strictly limited. A specially designed suit area may be provided in the facility. Personnel who enter this area wear a one-piece positive pressure suit that is ventilated by a life support system. The life support system is provided with alarms and emergency break-up breathing air tanks. Entry to this area is through an airlock fitted with air tight doors. A chemical shower is provided to decontaminate the surface of the suit before the worker leaves the area. The exhaust air form the suit area is filtered by two sets of HEPA filters installed in the series. A duplicate filtration unit, exhaust fan and an automatically starting emergency power source are provided. The air pressure within the suit area is lower than that of any adjacent area. Emergency lighting and communication systems are provided. All penetrations into the inner shell of the suit area are sealed. A double door autoclave is provided for decontamination of disposable waste materials from the suit area.

Chapter 3

Instruments of Microbiology Lab

Instruments of Microbiology Lab

The microbiology laboratory should contain the following basic instruments whether it is BSL 1 or 4, and it needs some basic infrastructure as shown in the layout.

The most commonly used instruments which are used in all the microbiology labs for some basic techniques like media preparation, aseptic transfer of culture, growth and storage of cultures. The other activities like morphological and biochemical characterization may vary on the requirements.

The most commonly employed instruments are

1. Weighing Balance
2. Autoclave
3. Hot air Oven
4. Laminar air flow Cabinet
5. Incubator
6. Refrigerator and Deep Freezer

Weighing Balance (Weighing Scales)

Weighing scales is a measuring instrument for determining the weight or mass of an object. The name scales derives from the pair of scales or dishes in which objects to be weighed and the weights / masses against which to weigh them are placed. Balance or scales can be calibrated to read in units of force (weight) such as Newtons, or in units of mass such as kilograms.

An analytical balance is commonly employed in most of the microbiology lab for weighing the chemicals and components of the media. It is a class of balance designed to measure small mass in the sub-milligram range. The measuring pan of an analytical balance (0.1 mg or better) is inside a transparent enclosure with doors so that dust does not collect and so any air currents in the room do not affect the balance's operation. This enclosure is often called a draft shield.

Currently the Electronic analytical scales are used to measure the force needed to counter the mass being measured rather than using actual masses. As such they must have calibration adjustments made to compensate for gravitational differences. They work on a principle that an electromagnet is used to generate a force to counter the sample being measured and outputs the result by measuring the force needed to achieve balance.

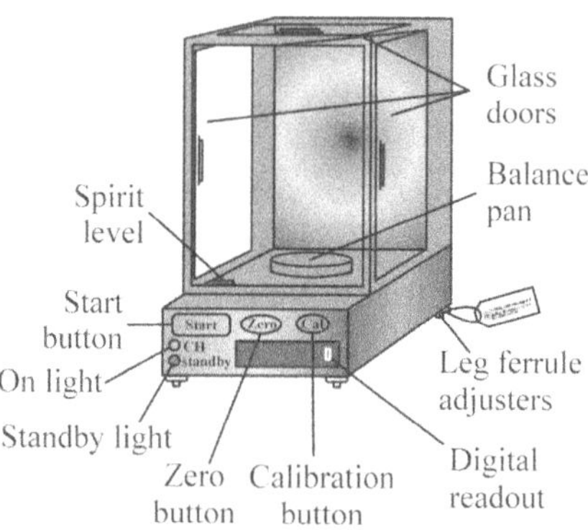

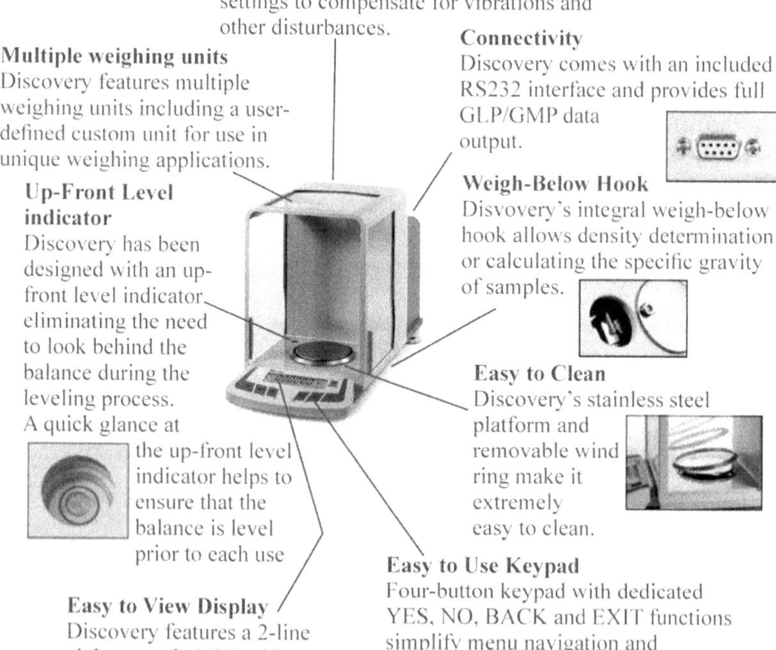

Fig. 3.1 Analytical balance.

Autoclave

It is a Greek word means auto-self, and clavis -key—a self-locking device. An autoclave is a device used to sterilize media, equipment and supplies by subjecting them to high pressure created by the saturated steam at 121 °C for around 15–20 minutes depending on the size of the load and the contents. It was invented by Charles Chamberland in 1879.

Autoclave in a microbiology laboratory is generally used for the sterilization of media, glassware's and waste materials.

It works on a basic principle of large pressure cooker; it operates by using steam under pressure in an insulated object as sterilizing agent. High pressures enable the steam to achieve high temperatures, which is needed to kill the microorganism. This high heating power of steam is based on latent heat of vaporization; it is the amount of heat required to convert boiling water to steam. For example, it takes 80 calories to make 1 liter of water boil, but 540 calories to convert that boiling water to steam. Therefore, steam at 100° C has almost seven times more heat than boiling water. Moreover Steam is able to penetrate objects with cooler temperatures because once the steam contacts a cooler surface; it immediately condenses to water, producing a concomitant 1,870 fold decrease in steam volume. This creates negative pressure at the point of condensation and draws more steam to the area. Condensations continue so long as the temperature of the condensing surface is less than that of steam; once temperatures equilibrate, a saturated steam environment is formed. Steam under pressure kills the microbial cells by breaking the intramolecular hydrogen bonds between proteins thereby causes coagulation of proteins which eventually causes halt to metabolic process. Autoclaves can be validated based on thermal death time (TDT) because it operates on a time/temperature relationship; increasing the temperature decreases TDT, and lowering the temperature increases TDT.

Table 3.1 Standard temperature and pressure of an autoclave processes

S. No	Temperature	Pressure
1	100°C	00 lb/in²
2	109°C	05 lb/in²
3	115°C	10 lb/in²
4	121°C	15 lb/in²
5	126°C	20 lb/in²
6	132°C	20 lb/in²

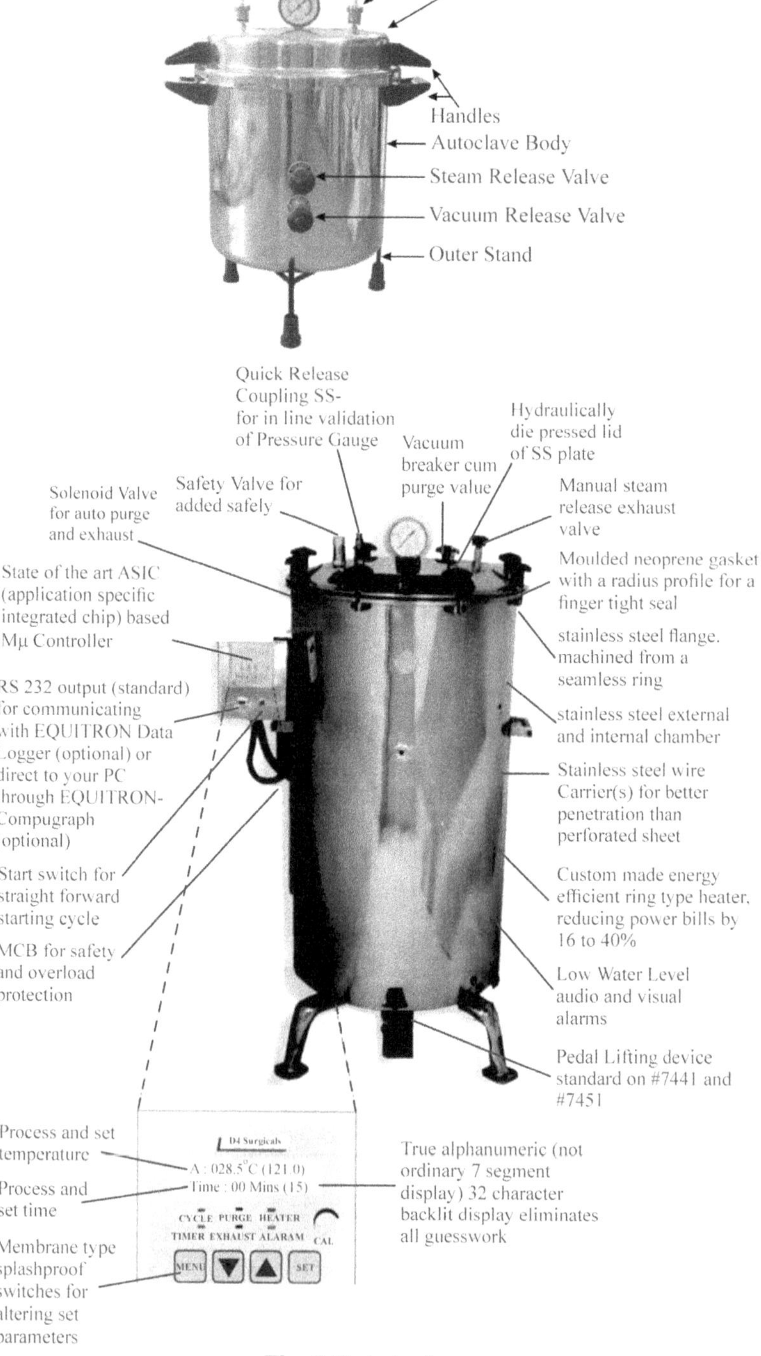

Fig. 3.2 Autoclave.

Hot Air Oven

This technique of sterilization was originally developed by Louis Pasteur. Hot air ovens are electrical devices used to sterilize articles like laboratory glasswares such as petri dishes and pipettes, oil and powders. which are thermo stable. Generally they can be operated from 50 to 300 °C (122 to 572 °F) with a thermostat controlling the temperature. The instrument contains double walled insulation which keeps the heat in and conserves energy, the inner layer being a poor conductor and outer layer being metallic. There is also an air filled space in between to aid insulation and an air circulating fan helps in uniform distribution of the heat. These are fitted with the adjustable wire mesh plated trays or aluminium trays and may have an on/off rocker switch, as well as indicators and controls for temperature and holding time. Temperature sensitive tapes or other devices like those using bacterial spores can be used to work as controls, to test for the efficacy of the device in every cycle.

A complete cycle involves heating the oven to the required temperature, maintaining that temperature for the proper time interval for that temperature, turning the machine off and cooling the articles in the closed oven till they reach room temperature. The standard settings for a hot air oven are: 1.5 to 2 hours at 160 °C (320 °F) and 6 to 12 minutes at 190 °C (374 °F) which does not include the time required to preheat the chamber before beginning the sterilization cycle. It kills the microorganism by coagulating the proteins.

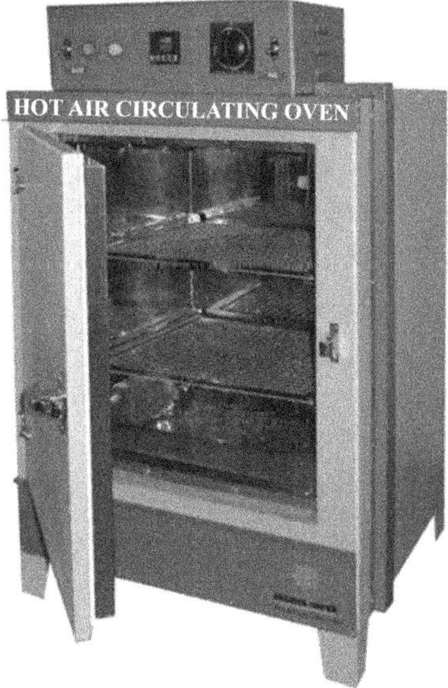

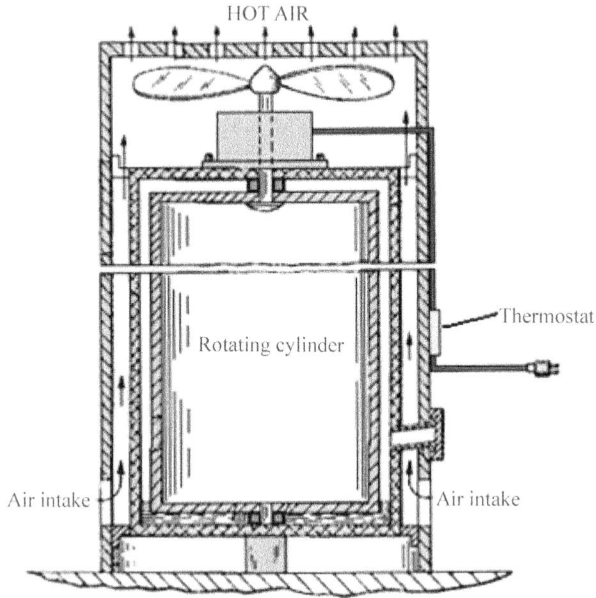

Fig. 3.3 Hot air oven.

Laminar Air Flow Cabinet

Laminar flow cabinet is an enclosed bench designed to prevent the contamination of biological samples from and to the external environment during the aseptic transfer of media or cultures for sub culturing activities. In the Laminar air flow Bench air is drawn through a HEPA (High Efficiency Particulate Absorption) qualify as HEPA by US government standards, an air filter must remove (from the air that passes through) 99.97% of particles that have a size of 0.3 micrometers or larger) filter and blown in a very smooth, laminar flow towards the user. The cabinet is usually made of stainless steel with no gaps or joints where spores might collect. Such hoods exist in both horizontal and vertical configurations, and there are many different types of cabinets with a variety of airflow patterns and acceptable uses.

Laminar flow cabinets may have a UV-C germicidal lamp (It has band at 253.7 nm and 185 nm due to the peak emission of the mercury within the lamp. 85 to 90% of the UV produced by these lamps is at 253.7 nm, while only 5 to 10 percent is at 185 nm) to sterilize the shell and contents.

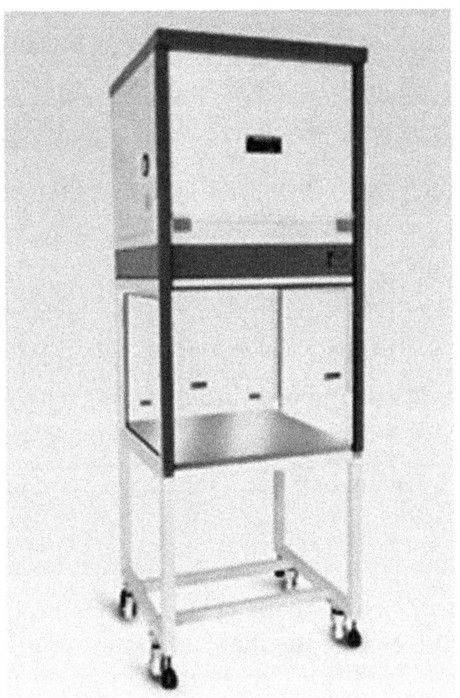

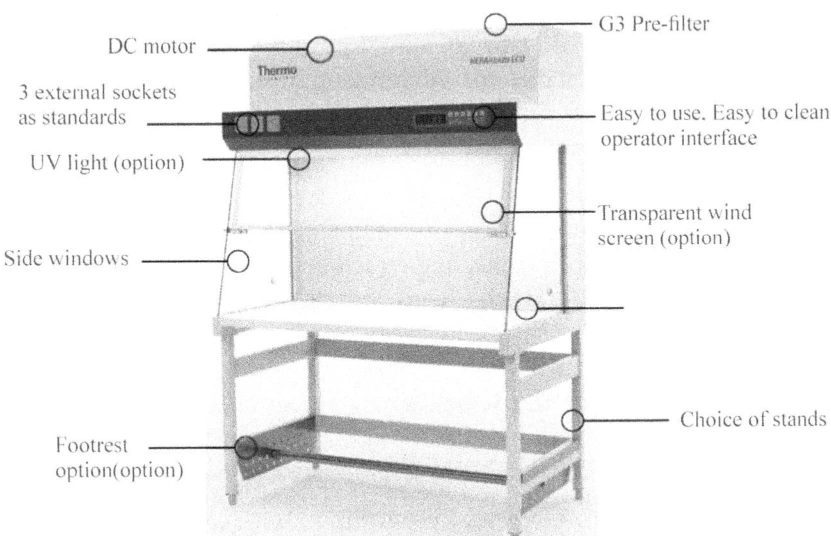

Fig. 3.4 Laminar air flow cabinet.

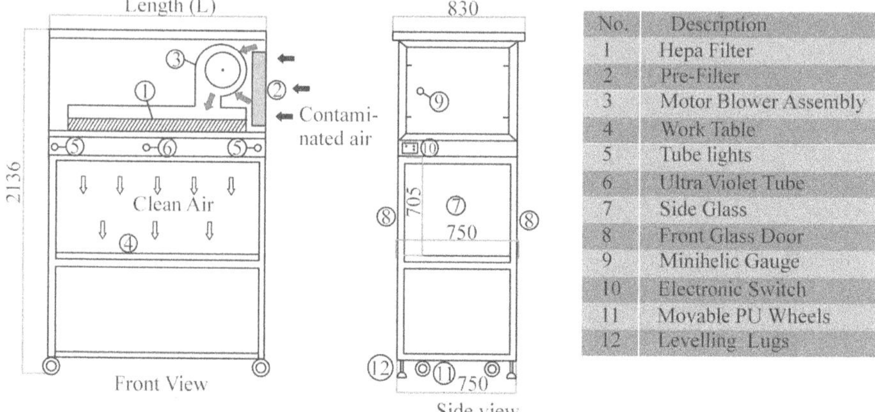

No.	Description
1	Hepa Filter
2	Pre-Filter
3	Motor Blower Assembly
4	Work Table
5	Tube lights
6	Ultra Violet Tube
7	Side Glass
8	Front Glass Door
9	Minihelic Gauge
10	Electronic Switch
11	Movable PU Wheels
12	Levelling Lugs

Fig. 3.5 Laminar air flow cabinet: front & side view.

Incubator

An incubator is a device used to grow and maintain microbiological cultures or cell cultures. The incubator maintains optimal temperature, humidity and other conditions such as the carbon dioxide (CO_2) and oxygen content of the atmosphere inside the chamber. The simplest incubators are insulated boxes with an adjustable heater, typically going up to 60 to 65 °C (140 to 150 °F). Some incubators include a timer with a programmable for cycle through different temperatures, humidity levels, etc. Incubators can vary in size from tabletop to units the size of small rooms.

The temperature of the incubator is controlled with the help of thermostat and the humidity is the major criteria because water is a major constituent of both broth and agar media. However, when media are incubated at temperatures used for bacterial cultivation, a large portion of water content can be lost through evaporation. Loss of water from media can be harmful to bacterial growth by increasing the solute concentration of the media which lyses bacterial cells. The humidity control can be achieved by placing a small, metal pan containing distilled water inside the incubator chamber.

The CO_2 incubators are usually equipped with flow meters, which monitor the flow of CO_2 in the unit. An indication of 0.5 liters per minute on the flow meter will provide approximately 5% CO_2 tension within the chamber. A CO_2 concentration of 3-10% is acceptable for most microorganisms requiring this environment.

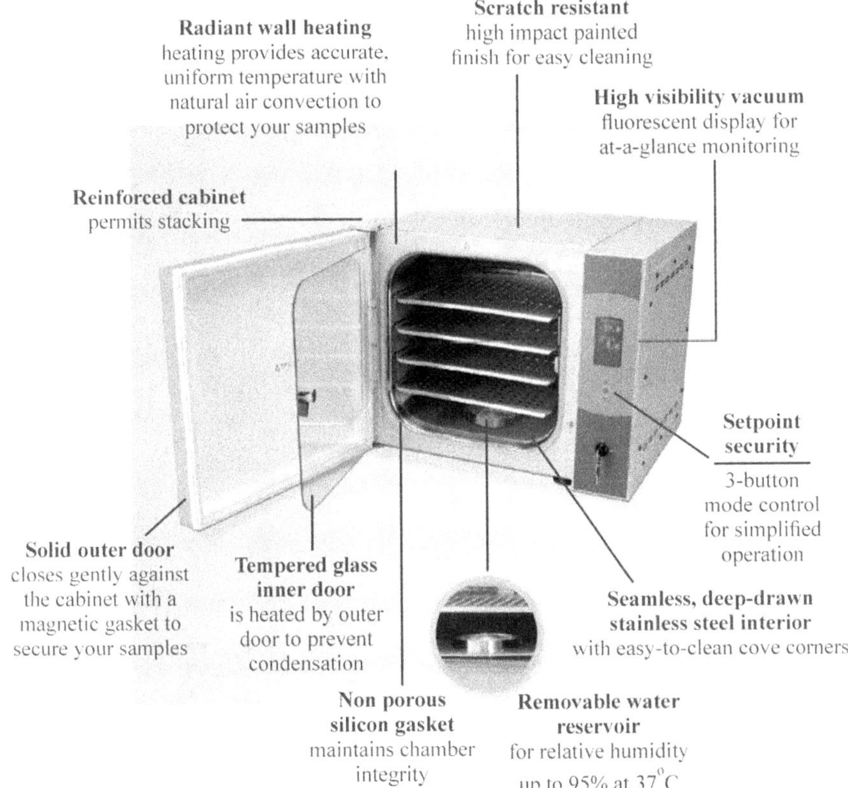

Fig. 3.6 Incubator.

Refrigerator and Deep Freezer

Refrigerator and deep freezer are used for storing the microbial cultures. A refrigerator consists of a thermally insulated compartment and a heat pump (mechanical, electronic, or chemical) that transfers heat from the inside of the fridge to its external environment so that the inside of the fridge is cooled to a temperature below the ambient temperature of the room.

A lower temperature in a confined volume lowers the reproduction rate of bacteria. Typically, medical refrigerator can be set at 40 F degrees to maintain temperatures in the range of 2° and 8°C degrees (35 F to 46 F degrees).

A similar device that maintains a temperature below the freezing point of water is called a freezer, a Deep freezer generally maintains temperature -18ºC and even lower.

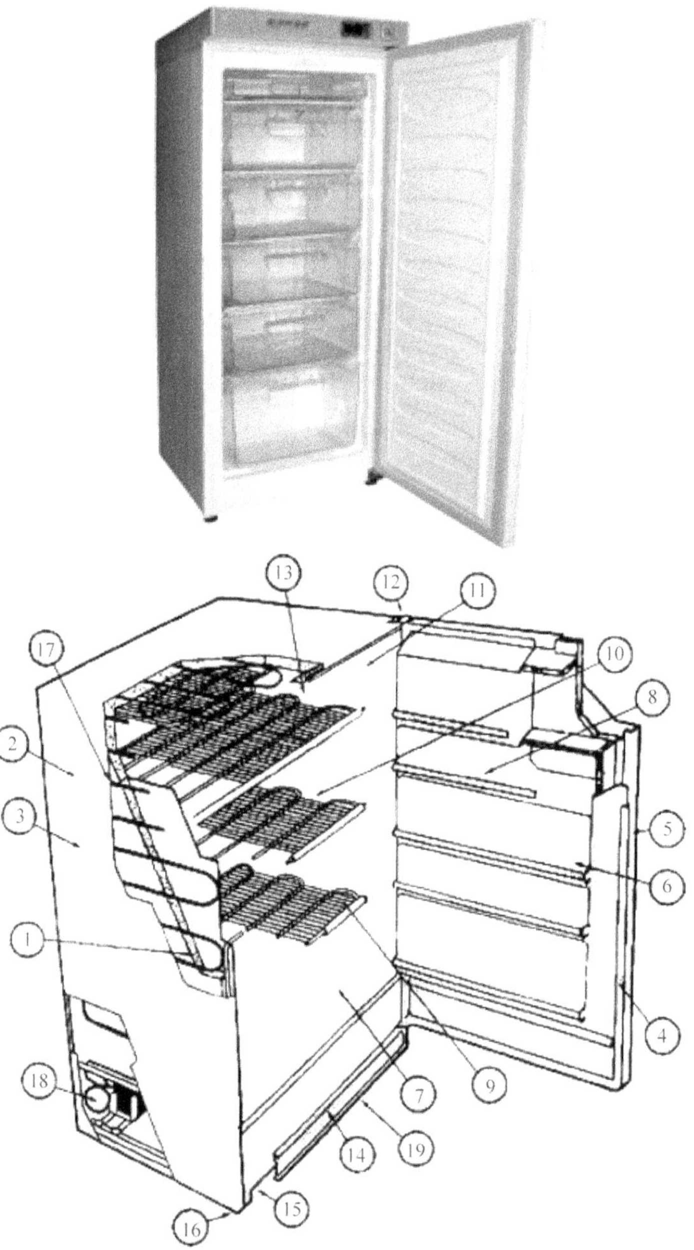

The parts of an upright home freezer: 1- polyurethane foam-insulation Cabinet, 2- wrap around steel cabinet, 3-baked on enamel finish, 4- magnetic door seal, 5- key ejecting lock, 6-bookshelf door storage, 7-slideoutbasket, 8 juice can shelf, 9- steel shelves, 10- fast two way freezing level, 11- temperature control knob, 12- door stops, 13-interior light, 14- power on light, 15 defrost water drain, 6- adjustable leveling legs, 17-coils welded to outer walls, 18-sealed compressor, and 19- RED

Fig. 3.7 Refrigerator.

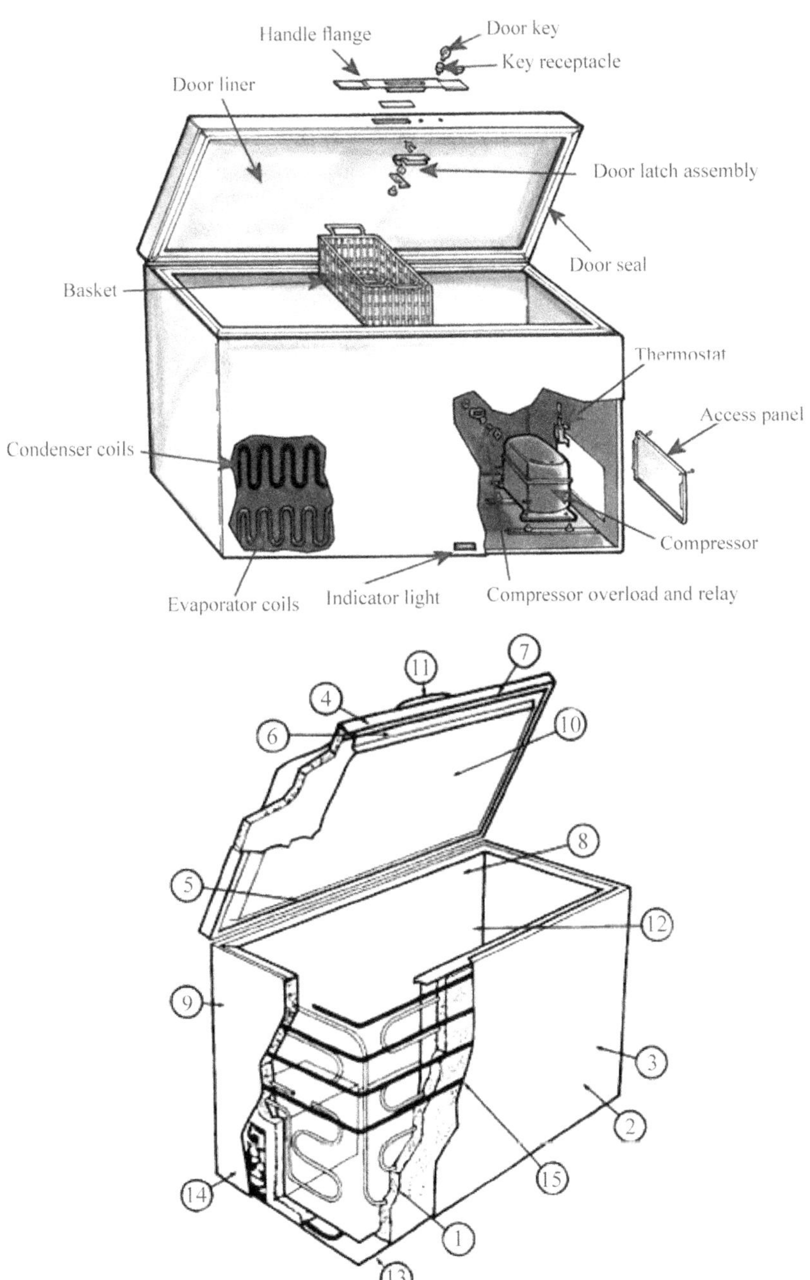

The parts of a chest type freezer: 1- polyurethane foam insulation, 2-wrap around steel cabinet, 3-baked on enamel finish, 4- self adjusting lid, 5-spring loaded hinges, 6-Vinyl lid gasket, 7- safely lock and self-ejecting key.8-lift out wire baskets, 9- temperature control knob, 10 automatic interior light, 11- power on light, 12 - vertical cabinet divider, 13-defrost water drain, 13- sealed compressor, and 15-wrap around condenser.

Fig. 3.8 Chest freezer.

PART - II

BASIC TECHNIQUES OF MICROBIOLOGY

Chapter 4

Optical Microscopy

Purpose

1. To understand the Historical Development and basic principle of working of microscope.
2. To become familiar with the operation of a light microscope.
3. To observe microorganisms using light microscopy.

Introduction

The discovery of microscope by Anton Van Leeuwenhoek was very basic model but the early microscopists had more problems because of optical aberration, blurred images, and poor lens design. Whereas the aberrations were partially corrected by the mid-nineteenth century with the introduction achromatic objectives by Lister and Amici, which reduced chromatic aberration and raised numerical apertures to around 0.65 for dry objectives and up to 1.25 for homogeneous immersion objectives. In 1886, Ernst Abbe's work with Carl Zeiss led to the production of apochromatic objectives based on sound optical principles and lens design. Latter in 1893 Professor August Köhler reported a method of illumination, which he developed to optimize photomicrography, had made the microscopists to take full advantage of the resolving power of Abbe's objectives.

Microscope

A microscope (Greek word meaning: micros-small and skope -to look) is an instrument used to see objects that are too small cannot be seen through naked eye. The microscope can be broadly classified based into optical and electron microscope based on the source of interaction with the sample to generate the image. The optical microscopes and transmission electron microscopes use the theory of lenses (optics for light microscopes and electromagnet lenses for electron microscopes) in order to magnify the image generated by the passage of a wave (electromagnetic radiation in optical microscopes and electron beams in electron microscopes) transmitted through the sample, or reflected by the sample.

Principle of Microscopy

Microscope works on two basic principle; magnification and resolution. The smaller objects can be magnified with help of magnifying glass which when put between the eye and the object makes everything appear larger. However, there is a limit to this method: a magnification of more than 8-fold or 10-fold is not possible because the image started getting distortion after certain magnification, so there is need of resolution or minimum resolvable distance which is the minimum distance between distinguishable objects in an image.

Magnification of Microscope

In microscope several lenses can be arranged one behind the other for the maximum magnifications up to 2000X. The classic microscope magnifies in two steps: The objective produces a magnified image of the object called as intermediate image plane, and the eyepiece magnifies the intermediate image in the same way as a magnifier and produces the final image.

The light is emitted from an object is processed by a group of lenses for magnification. The eyepiece, in turn, serves as a magnifying glass to make this small intermediate image appear even more magnified to the eye.

So the total magnification can be calculated as

Total Magnification = Objective Magnification × Eyepiece magnification

For example if an objective lens is 100X and the eyepiece lens is 20X then the magnification of the object is $100 \times 20 = 2000X$.

Resolution of Microscope

Resolving power or resolution can be defined as the limit up to which two small objects are still seen separately in a microscope. A certain distance d_0 exists where this limit is reached. It can also be calculated theoretically as

$$d_0 = \frac{1.22\,\lambda}{N.A_{obj} + N.A_{cond}} = \frac{\lambda}{2N.A}$$

Where as the λ = wavelength of light for optical microscope (400 to 700nm), N.A is numerical aperture. The higher the aperture of the objective (N.A. Obj.) and of the condenser (N.A. cond.), the smaller d_0 will be. A short wavelength is also beneficial for the resolving power.

The numerical aperture (N.A) can be defined as this is a measure of the solid angle covered by an objective, which can be calculated as

Numerical Aperture (N.A) = n. sin α

α is half the opening angle of the objective and n is the refractive index of the immersion medium used between the objective and the object (n = 1 for air; n = 1.51 for oil or glass).

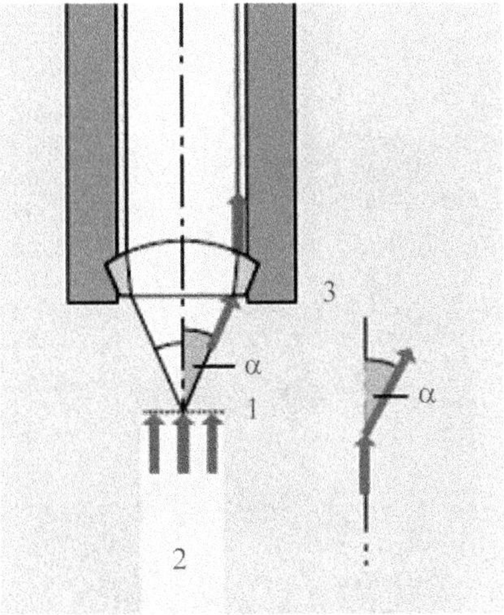

Fig. 4.1 Resolution of microscope.

1: is a small object (glass slide with specimen) are viewed through the microscope, 2: is the incident light and 3; is the objective of the microscope which collect as much of this diffracted light as possible.

The following table shows the values for the resolution resulting from the calculation for some objectives. The distance d_0 is referred to the specimen and, when multiplied by the magnification, results in the point distance D_0 in the intermediate image (for green light λ = 550 nm).

S. No.	Objective/ NA	d_0 (μm)	D_0 (μm)
1	5x / 0.15	2.2	11.2
2	10x / 0.30	1.1	11.2
3	20x / 0.50	0.7	13.4
4	40x / 0.75	0.45	17.9
5	40x / 1.30 Oil	0.26	10.3
6	100x / 1.30 Oil	0.26	25.8

Handling of Microscope

A typical optical microscope and their parts has shown in the figure and the pathway of light from the source to the eyepiece had been illustrated in the diagram.

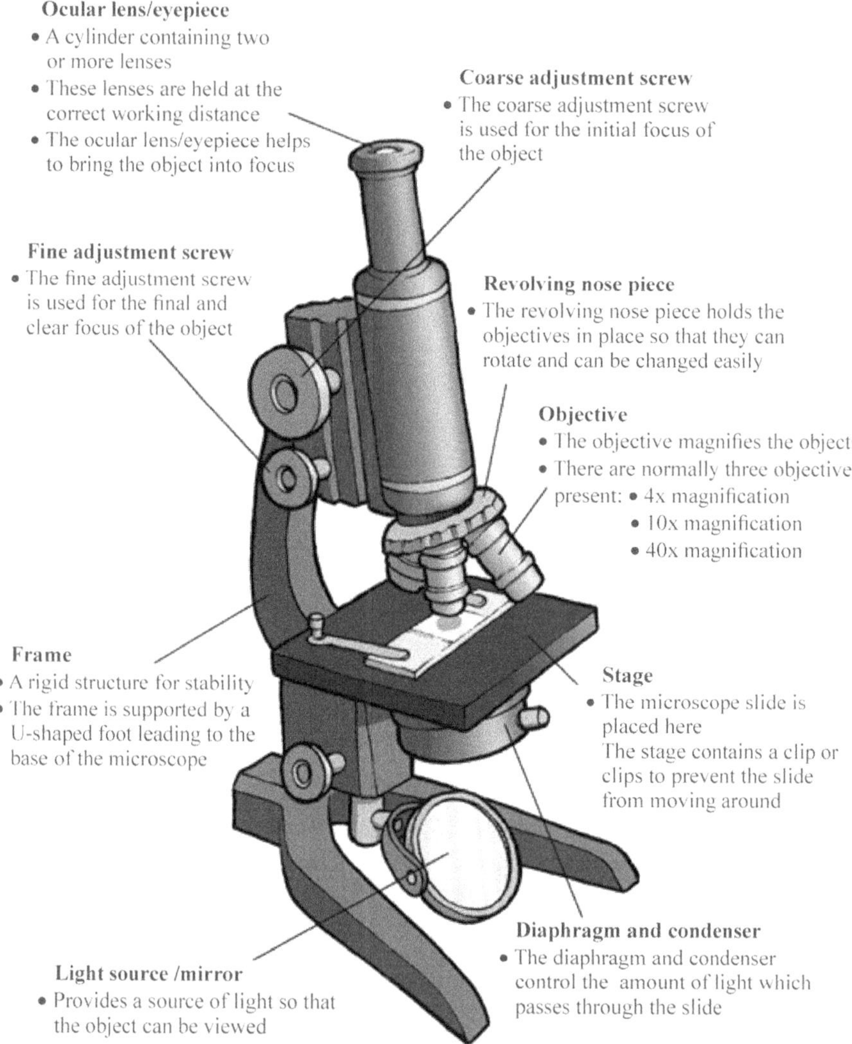

Fig. 4.2 Compound microscope.

Working with Microscope

1. Switch on the light source and hold the paper strip to check the visibility of the light above the luminous-field diaphragm in the

stand. Normally, however, you will see a spot of light on the paper (If everything remains dark, line plug, illuminator and fuse of the power unit must be checked and the necessary changes made).

2. Completely open the luminous-field diaphragm until the spot of light on the paper reaches its maximum diameter.

3. Now hold the paper strip between the sample and the objective. Fully open the aperture diaphragm of the condenser. The small light spot on the paper will then show its maximum brightness.

4. The height of the condenser can be adjusted with the help of condenser drive. Set the condenser height in such a way that its front lens is approx. 1-3 mm away from the sample from below. Now a day's modern instrument have an adjustable stop screw allowing the top position of the condenser to be fixed.

5. Light should now already be discernable in the eyepieces. If it is very bright, reduce the brightness until you find it comfortable to work with. Then set the interpupillary distance via the folding bridge of the binocular tube. The correct setting is reached when you see one light circle instead of two.

6. Now look into the microscope and carefully move the stage, including the sample, up and down until you see the details as sharply as possible.

7. If you will not see a perfect image because the illumination is not correct than narrow the luminous-field diaphragm and move the condenser carefully up and down via the condenser drive until you see a sharp image of the luminous-field diaphragm, or at least a piece of it in the edge.

8. Adjust the coarse and fine adjustments until you get a clear image.

9. In practical microscopy, nicely stained samples which are easy to view in simple brightfield. Unstained samples, such as bacteria or living cell cultures, absorb practically no light and are barely or not at all visible in brightfield, even in a well-aligned microscope.

10. If you are using the 100X (oil) objective lens than place a drop of cidarwood oil between the object and the objective lens and the fine adjustment is made until a clear image is observed.

11. After viewing the image the slide is removed and discarded in proper manner and the microscope should be covered when it was in ideal condition.

Observing the Microorganism

Material Required

1. Microscope
2. Lens paper
3. Prepared slides of various cultures of microorganisms.
4. Immersion oil

Observation

1. Calculate the total magnification for each of the objective lenses on your microscope.

Objective lens power	X	Ocular lens power	= Total magnification

2. Look at a prepared slide. Draw a picture of what you observe. Be sure to note the magnification at which you did the drawing

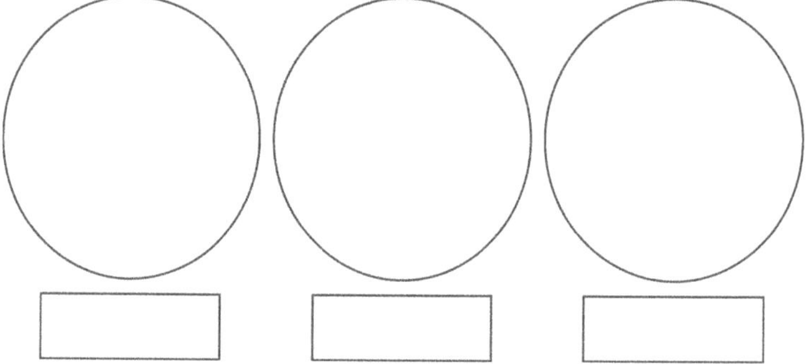

Chapter 5

Preparation and Sterilization of Media

Purpose

1. To understand the nutritional requirement of bacteria and different types of media.
2. To prepared and sterilize nutrient broth and nutrient agar media for 100mL.
3. To prepare Agar slant, Agar deep tube and Agar cake.

Introduction

All living cells in this world requires nutrients for their survival, growth and energy production similarly the microorganisms are extraordinarily diverse in their requirements of nutrients for their growth. If we understand the nutritional needs of any microorganism we can cultivate the microorganism in the laboratory.

Nutritional Requirement

Based on the nutritional requirement of the microorganism it can be classified into major nutrients, minor nutrients and trace elements.

Major Nutrients (C, H, O, N, S and P)

The major nutrients are required in large quantities and it is needed to meet its growth and energy production. The carbon, Hydrogen, Oxygen are the major building block of the organism and they are principle energy requirements. Based on the carbon source the microbes can be classified as **Autotrophs and Heterotrophs. Autotrophs** are organisms that are able to use inorganic carbon dioxide as their sole carbon source for the biosynthesis of macromolecules. **Heterotrophs**, require organic carbon for biosynthesis.

Autotrophs can be further broken down into two categories: the **chemoautotrophs** derive energy from the oxidation of inorganic compounds such as iron, hydrogen sulfide and hydrogen gas. **Photoautotrophs**, such as the **cyanobacteria**, convert light energy into chemical energy.

Heterotrophic organisms can also be divided into two major subgroups. **Photoheterotrophs**, use organic carbon sources for biosynthesis but use light energy to produce ATP (photosynthesis). **Chemoheterotrophs**, use organic compounds such as sugars, proteins and lipids as their source of energy.

As chemoheterotrophs are more abundant and easier to work with, one usually works with these organisms in a typical teaching laboratory setting.

Generally the Oxygen and hydrogen will be obtained from water and from carbon source itself.

Nitrogen is the basic component of cell and nucleic acid. It is obtained from inorganic source like nitrates, nitrites and ammonium salts and also from organic source from amino acids.

Sulphur is necessary for the synthesis of certain amino acids like cysteine, cystine and methionine and it is obtained either from elemental sulphur or from inorganic sources.

Phosphorous is supplied from phosphates and it is necessary for Nucleic acid synthesis and ATP production.

Minor Nutrients

These are required in low concentration basically to maintain the cell potential difference and as co factors for biochemical pathways. These include majorly the metal ions like potassium, calcium, magnesium and iron.

Trace Elements

These are required at very low concentration and generally available as contaminant with other constituents, these include Zinc, Copper, manganese, molybdenum, nickel, Boron and cobalt called as trace elements.

Media

Media is the nutritional composition required by the microorganism which can be satisfactorily cultivated in the laboratory environment.

The media in a laboratory setting may be classified as **defined** or **complex (undefined)**.

Defined media: A defined media is a media in which all of the constituents and the amounts of these constituents are known. Defined media typically supports a narrower range of heterotrophic microorganisms. Defined media typically consist of salts and a carbon source in the form of glucose. Depending on the fastidiousness of an organism, these media can be supplemented with vitamins, nucleic acids, cofactors and amino acids.

Complex media: Complex media are composed of extracts from plants, animals or yeast and therefore are rich in nutrients. Such media is complex because the precise individual components of these media are unknown; however, as these media contain a wide range of nutrients that are well above the minimal nutritional requirements of the organism being cultured, these media support the growth of a wide range of organisms.

Material Required:

Chemicals Required:

1. Peptone
2. Sodium chloride
3. Beef extract
4. Yeast extract

Glassware Required:

1. 250 mL Conical Flask
2. 100 mL Measuring Cylinder
3. 100 mL Beaker
4. Absorbent Cotton

Equipments required

1. Autoclave
2. Hot air oven
3. Laminar airflow cabinet
4. Incubator

Composition of Nutrient Broth Media – 1000 mL

S. No.	Chemical	Quantity gm/L	Quantity Needed for 100ml
1	Peptone	5.0	
2	Beef Extract	1.5	
3	Yeast Extract	1.5	
4	Sodium Chloride	5.0	
5	Distilled water	1000 mL	
	pH adjusted to 7.4 ± 0.2		

Composition of Nutrient Agar Medium – 1000 mL

S. No.	Chemical	Quantity gm/L	Quantity Needed for 100ml
1	Peptone	5.0	
2	Beef Extract	1.5	
3	Yeast Extract	1.5	
4	Sodium Chloride	5.0	
5	Agar Agar	2 % (20.0)	
6	Distilled water	1000 mL	
	pH adjusted to 7.4 ± 0.2		

Procedure

Preparation and Sterilization of Nutrient Broth Medium

1. Accurately weigh all the ingredients and add to a 250mL conical flask.

2. Add 50ml of water and mix it to dissolve and add rest 50 mL of distilled water.

3. Adjust the pH with 0.1N NaOH or 0.1N H_2SO_4 to pH 7.4 by means of adding drop wise and stirring well. if the initial pH is acidic, add 0.1N NaOH and if it is alkaline add 0.1N H_2SO_4

4. Add the media in to the test tube and plug with cotton.

5. Place all the test tube in a beaker and sterilize in autoclave at 121ºC for 15 min.

Preparation and Sterilization of Nutrient Agar Medium

1. Accurately weigh all the ingredients except agar-agar and add to a 250 mL conical flask.

2. Add 50 mL of water and mix it to dissolve

3. Add agar-agar and heat in water bath for 30 minutes until it get dissolved and add rest 50 mL of distilled water.

4. Adjust the pH with 0.1N NaOH or 0.1N H_2SO_4 to pH 7.4 by means of adding drop wise and stirring well. if the initial pH is acidic, add 0.1N NaOH and if it is alkaline add 0.1N H_2SO_4

5. Plug cotton to the conical flask and sterilize in autoclave at 121ºC for 15 min.

Preparation of Nutrient Agar Slant, Deep tube and Cake

1. Plug the empty test tube with cotton and place all the test tube in a beaker.

2. Sterilize the test tube in autoclave at 121ºC for 15 min.

3. Sterilize the washed petridish in hot air oven at 200ºC for 2 hrs.

4. After sterilization bring all the test tube, petri-dish and Nutrient agar medium in the laminar air flow cabinet.

5. Aseptically transfer the Nutrient agar medium from conical flask while it is hot (around 60ºC, if it reached below 45 ºC it gets solidified - before that complete all the process) to 1/3rd of the test tube and keep in slant position and allow it to solidify – Nutrient agar slant.

6. Similarly aseptically transfer the Nutrient agar medium from conical flask while it is hot to 1/3rd of the test tube and keep in straight position in a test tube stand and allow it to solidify – Nutrient agar Deep tube.

7. For the preparation of Nutrient agar cake - Aseptically transfer the Nutrient agar medium from conical flask while it is hot to the petridish and allow it to solidify. (take care that the water droplets won't be present at the top of the petridish or no air bubble is entrapped while pouring in the petridish)

Observation

Report

Chapter 6

Aseptic Transfer of Bacterial Culture

Purpose

1. To understand the aseptic transfer of bacterial culture or sub culturing process.
2. To perform the technique of aseptic removal and transfer of microorganism to freshly prepared media.

Principle

In the microbiology laboratory routinely the microorganism had been transfer to fresh medium form the older culture, this process is called as sub culturing. This procedure is very important and basic for all the microbiology and pathology laboratories for maintaining the cultures. Since the microorganism is present everywhere like lab equipments, personal, lab benches etc, so there is a need of aseptic transfer during the sub culturing process to avoid these external contaminations.

Sub culturing involves three steps:

1. Transferring of the organism from an old culture to a new culture medium.
2. Incubation at 37°C for 24 hours.
3. Preservation of the culture.

Sub culturing is done as the accumulation of toxins and exhaustion of nutrients may occur in the old medium and the organism may get killed,

The organisms have to be in constant supply of nutrition. They cannot be kept on the same medium for more than 3 weeks as the microorganism may lose some of their inherent properties or may undergo mutation or may get contaminated with other organisms due to aging.

Sub culturing is always done on a solid nutrient agar medium either by streaking or stabbing method.

The aseptic process of culture transfer is generally carried out in Laminar airflow cabinet as discussed in chapter 3.

Material Required

Instrument: Laminar airflow cabinet, Bunsen burner, inoculation loop and needle, and glassware marking pen.

Fresh media: One nutrient broth test-tube, one nutrient agar slant and one nutrient agar deep tube.

Culture: 24 hr nutrient broth culture of *E. coli.*

Procedure

Sterilization of Laminar Airflow Cabinet

1. The working platform of the laminar airflow cabinet is cleaned with ethanol using cotton.
2. The UV light is switched ON and allows sterilizing for 15 minutes (during the process close the cabinet glass door and keep away from the direct contact because UV radiation cause cancer).
3. Switch OFF the UV light and ON the Fluorescence light.

Aseptic Transfer

Follow the procedure as illustrated in the Figure 6.1.

1. First the hands should be sterilized with ethanol by washing and allow to dry completely, place the Bunsen burner at the center of the working platform and illuminate it.
2. Keep three test tube stands; one contains the old culture, second contain the fresh media and an empty test tube stand to place the transferred culture.
3. Label the fresh media test tube with organism name, date of inoculation and initial of inoculator.
4. Place the tubes in the palm of your hand, secure with your thumb, and separate to form a V shape as shown in the illustration.
5. Sterilize the inoculating needle or loop by showing in the blue flame until the entire wire is red hot.
6. With the sterile loop or needle in hand, uncap the tubes.
7. Flame the necks of the tubes by rapidly passing them through the flame once.
8. Transfer the microorganism from the old culture to the new media with the help of sterile inoculation loop or needle.
9. Flame the necks once again by rapidly passing them through the flame.
10. Recap the tubes.

11. Reflame the inoculating loop or needle to red hot once again to sterilize.

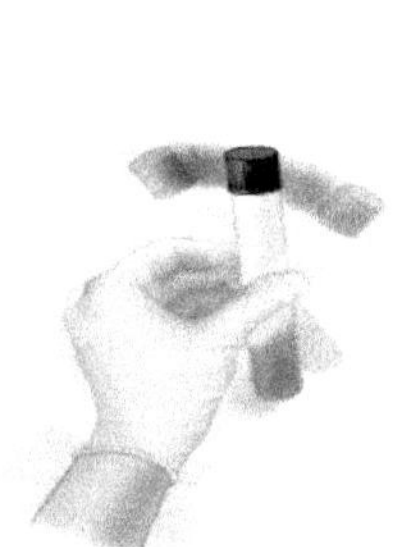

(1) Shake the culture tube from side to side to suspend organisms. Do not moisten cap on tube.

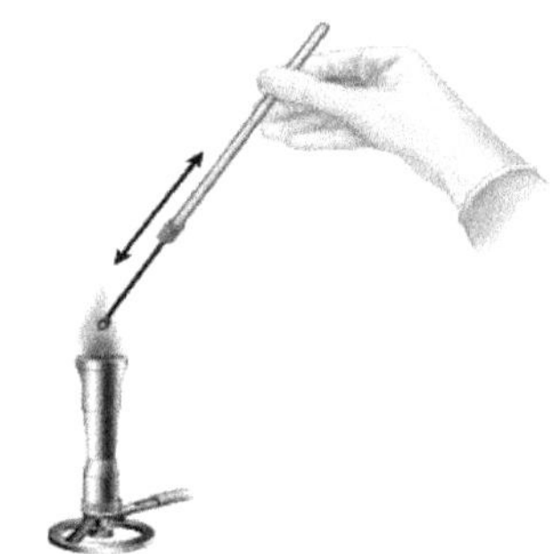

(2) Heat loop and wire to red-hot. Flame the handle slightly also.

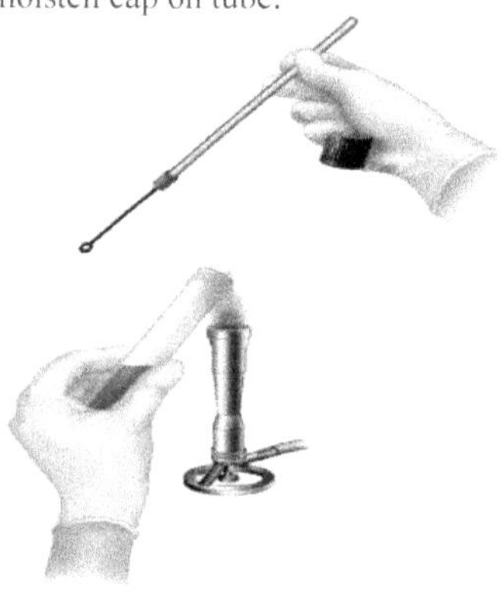

(3) Remove the cap and flame the neck of the tube. Do not place the cap down on the table.

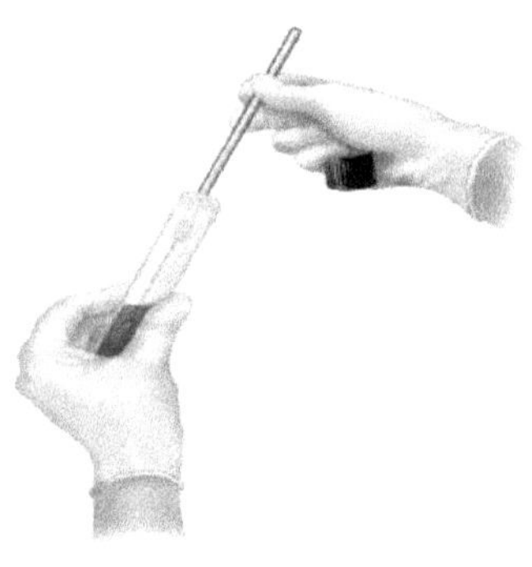

(4) After allowing the loop to cool for at least 5 seconds, remove a loopful of organisms. Avoid touching the side of the tube.

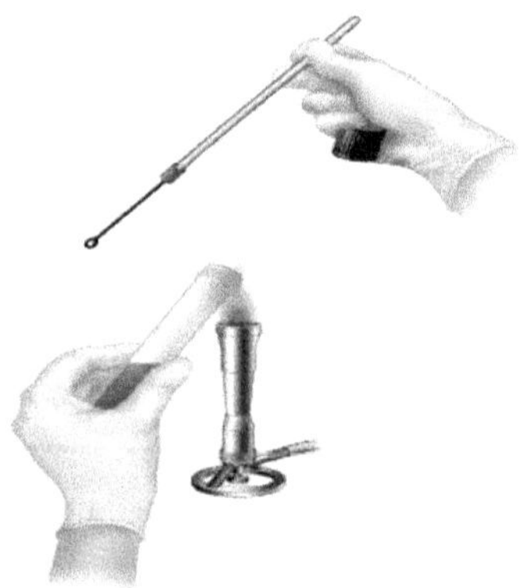

(5) Flame the mouth of the culture tube again.

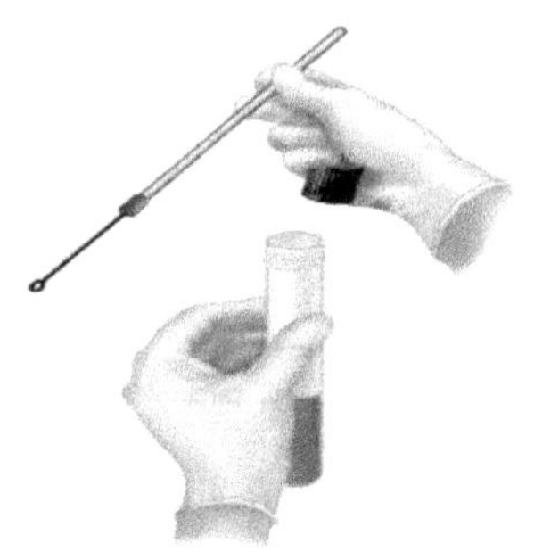

(6) Return the cap to the tube and place the tube in a test-tube rack.

Fig. 6.1 Aseptic transfer technique.

1. Keep the test tubes in respective stands.
2. Wash the hand with ethanol once again.
3. Repeat the process of sterilization of laminar airflow cabinet before leaving the aseptic room.

Report:

PART - III

MORPHOLOGICAL CHARACTERIZATION OF BACTERIA

Chapter 7

Colony Characteristics of Bacteria

Purpose

1. To perform the spread plate technique.
2. To study the colony characteristic of given sample of micro-organism after performing spread plate technique.

Principle

In natural habitats, bacteria usually grow together in populations containing a number of species. In order to adequately study and characterize an individual bacterial species, we have to isolate the organism in **pure culture.**

The **spread plate technique** is an easy, direct way of achieving this isolation process. In this technique, a small volume of dilute bacterial mixture containing 100 to 200 cells or less is transferred to the center of an agar plate and is spread evenly over the surface with a sterile, L-shaped glass rod. The glass rod is normally sterilized by dipping in alcohol and flamed to burn off the alcohol. After incubation, some of the dispersed cells develop into isolated colonies.

A **colony** is a large number of bacterial cells on solid medium, which is visible to the naked eye as a discrete entity. In this procedure, one assumes that a colony is derived from one cell and therefore represents a clone of a pure culture. After incubation, the general form of the colony and the shape of the edge or margin can be determined by looking down at the top of the colony. The nature of the colony elevation is apparent when viewed from the side as the plate is held at eye level.

These variations are illustrated in Figure 7.1. After a well-isolated colony has been identified, it can then be picked up and streaked onto a fresh medium to obtain a pure culture.

Materials Required

Instrument: Bunsen burner, inoculating loop, 95% ethyl alcohol, L-shaped glass rod, 500-ml beaker, pipettes with pipettor and glassware marking pen.
Culture: 24- to 48-hour soil culture.

Procedure

1. With a glassware marking pen, label the bottom of the agar medium plates with the name of the soil to be inoculated, initial, and date of inoculation.

2. Pipette 0.1 mL of the soil sample onto the center of a agar plate

3. Dip the L-shaped glass rod into a beaker of ethanol and then tap the rod on the side of the beaker to remove any excess ethanol.

4. Briefly pass the ethanol-soaked spreader through the flame to burn off the alcohol and allow it to cool inside the lid of a sterile petri plate.

5. Spread the bacterial sample evenly over the agar surface with the sterilized spreader, making sure the entire surface of the plate has been covered. Also make sure you do not touch the edge of the plate as shown in the figure.

6. Immerse the spreader in ethanol, tap on the side of the beaker to remove any excess ethanol, and reflame.

7. Invert the plates and incubate for 24 to 48 hours at room temperature or 30°C.

8. After incubation, measure some representative colonies and carefully observe their morphology **(Bacterial Colony Characteristics on Agar Media as Seen with the Naked Eye).**

9. The characteristics of bacterial colonies are show in the figure.

10. Record your results in the report.

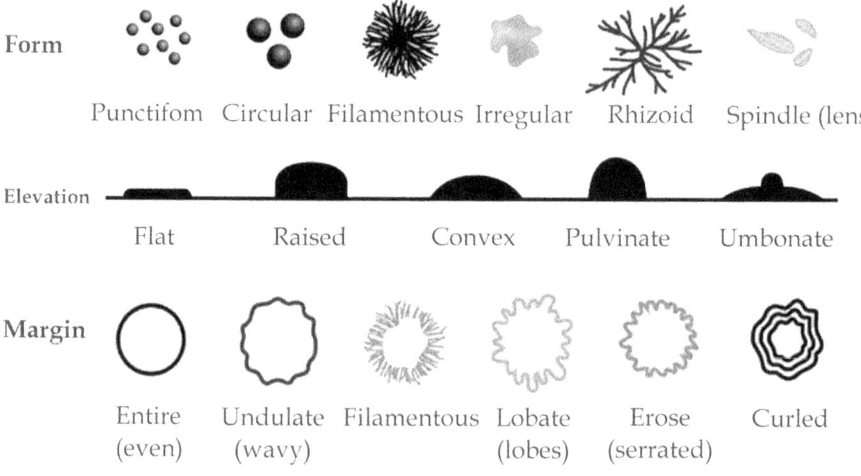

Fig. 7.1 Colony characteristics of bacteria.

Observation: Morphological colony characteristics

S. No	Characteristics	Observation	Diagram
1	Color or pigmentation		
2	Appearance		
3	Texture		
4	Form		
5	Elevation		
6	Margin		

Report

Chapter 8

Preparation of Specimen for Staining

Object

1. To perform the bacterial smear preparation by heat fixation technique.

Principle

A **bacterial smear** is a dried preparation of bacterial cells on a clean glass slide. a proper bacterial smear preparation can be obtained by

1. The bacteria should be used in such concentration that they are adequately separated from one another are evenly spread out on the slide.

2. After the fixation the bacterial smear should not washed off the slide during staining procedure and

3. During the heat fixation the bacterial form should not be distorted.

In making a smear, bacteria from either a broth culture or an agar slant or plate may be used. If a slant or plate is used, a *small* amount of bacterial growth is transferred to a drop of water on a glass slide **(Figure 8.1 a)** and mixed. The mixture is then spread out evenly over a large area on the slide **(Figure 8.1 b).** If the medium is liquid, place one or two loops of the medium directly on the slide **(Figure 8.1 c)** and spread the bacteria over a large area **(Figure 8.1 d).** Allow the slide to air dry at room temperature **(Figure 8.1 e).**

After the smear is dry, the heat fixation is done by gentle passing the slide several times through the hot portion of the flame of a Bunsen burner **(Figure 8.1 f).** Most bacteria can be **fixed** to the slide and killed in this way without serious distortion of cell structure.

Material Required

Instrument required: Clean microscope slides, bibulous paper, inoculating loop and needle, sterile distilled water, Bunsen burner and slide holder.

Culture: 24- to 48-hr broth or agar slants of *E. coli.*

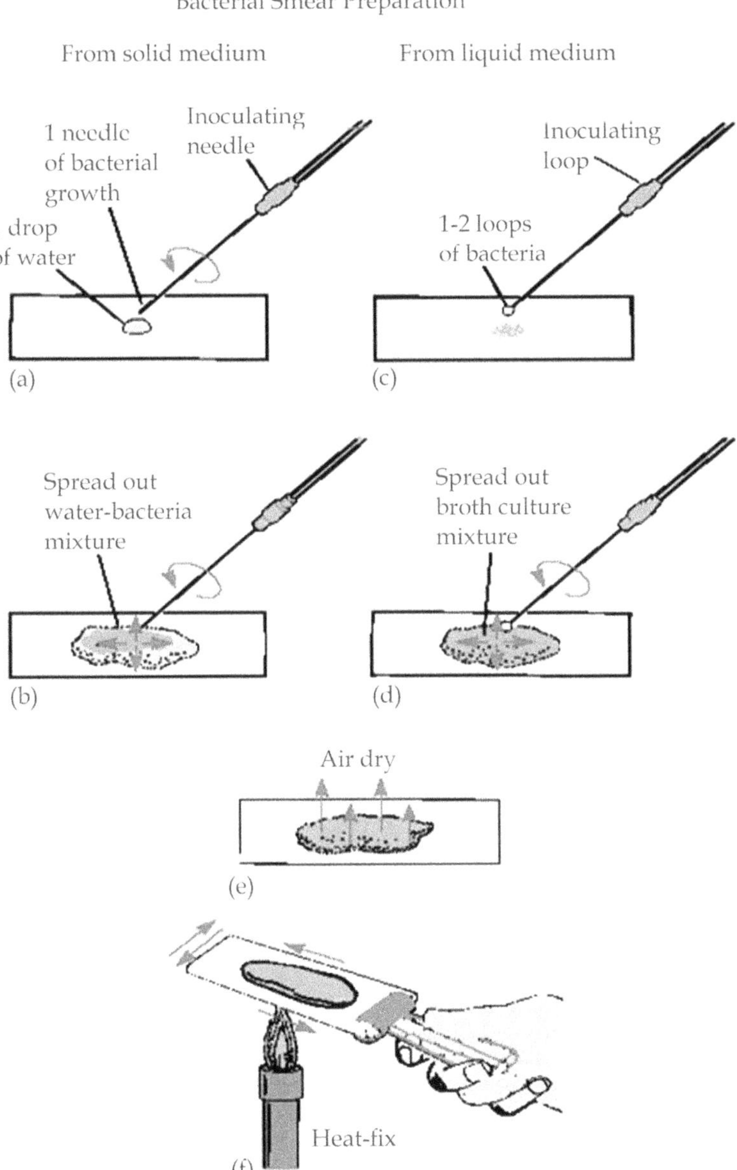

Fig. 8.1 Bacterial smear preparation.

Procedure

1. With the glassware marking pen, mark the name of the bacterial culture in the far left corner of the glass slides.
2. For the broth culture, shake the culture tube and, with an inoculating loop, aseptically (*see figure* 8.1) transfer 1 to 2 loopfuls of bacteria to the center of the slide. Spread this out to about a d-inch area.
3. When preparing a smear from a slant or plate, place a loopful of water in the center of the slide. With the inoculating needle, aseptically pick up a *very small* amount of culture and mix into the drop of water. Spread this out as above.
4. Allow the slide to air dry, or place it on a slide warmer (figure 8.1).
5. Pass the slide through a Bunsen burner flame three times to heat-fix and kill the bacteria.

Observation

Report

Chapter 9

Simple Staining

Object

1. To perform the simple staining.

Principle

In simple staining a single stain or dye is used to create contrast between the bacteria and its background. It is a very simple technique to study the cell shape, size, and arrangement. In this technique the heat fixed smear is flood with desired stain for the proper amount of time and then excess of stain is washed with water for a few seconds, finally, blots it dried and observed under the microscope.

Basic dyes such as **crystal violet** (20 to 30 seconds staining time), **carbolfuchsin** (5 to 10 seconds staining time), or **methylene blue** (1 minute staining time) are often used. Once bacteria have been properly stained, it is usually an easy matter to discern their overall shape. Bacterial morphology is usually uncomplicated and limited to one of a few variations.

Material Required

Instrument required: Clean microscope slides, bibulous paper, inoculating loop and needle, sterile distilled water, methylene blue, crystal violet (1% aqueous solution), Bunsen burner, slide rack, Microscope, immersion oil, lens paper and lens cleaner.

Culture: 24- to 48-hr broth or agar slants of *E. coli* and *Pseudomonas aureginousa.*

Procedure (See illustration also)

1. Prepare the smear for *E. coli* and *Pseudomonas aureginousa* in two separate glass slide as discussed in chapter 8.
2. Place the two fixed smears on a slide rack over a sink or other suitable receptacle.

3. Stain one slide with alkaline methylene blue for one minutes and another slide with crystal violet for 20 to 30 seconds.

4. Wash excess of stain with water for a few seconds.

5. Blot slide dry with bibulous paper (do not rub the smear when drying the slide because this will remove the stained bacteria).

6. Examine under the microscope at 20X, 40X and 100X (oil immersion) lens.

7. Record the reading. Common bacterial shapes also given in the figure 9.2.

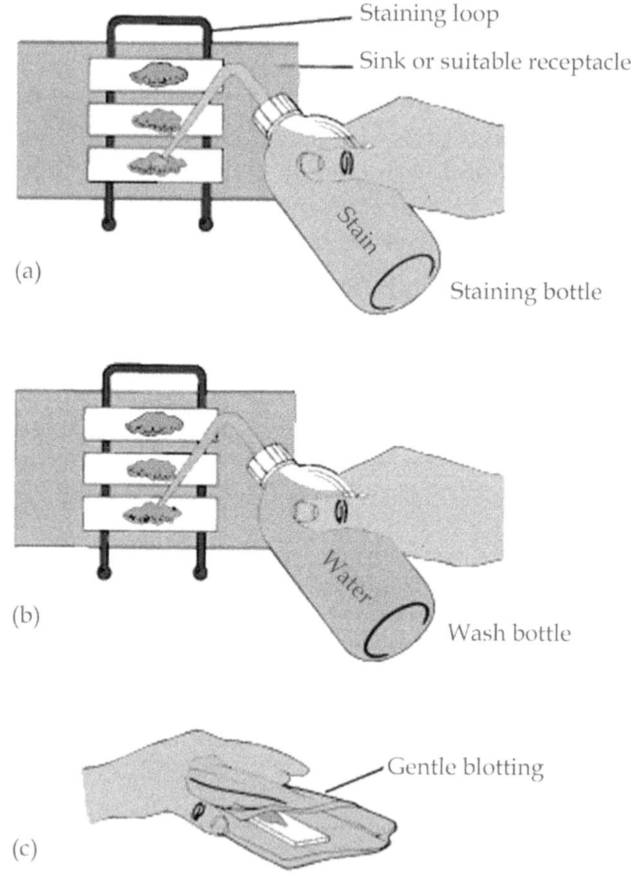

Fig. 9.1 Simple staining procedure.

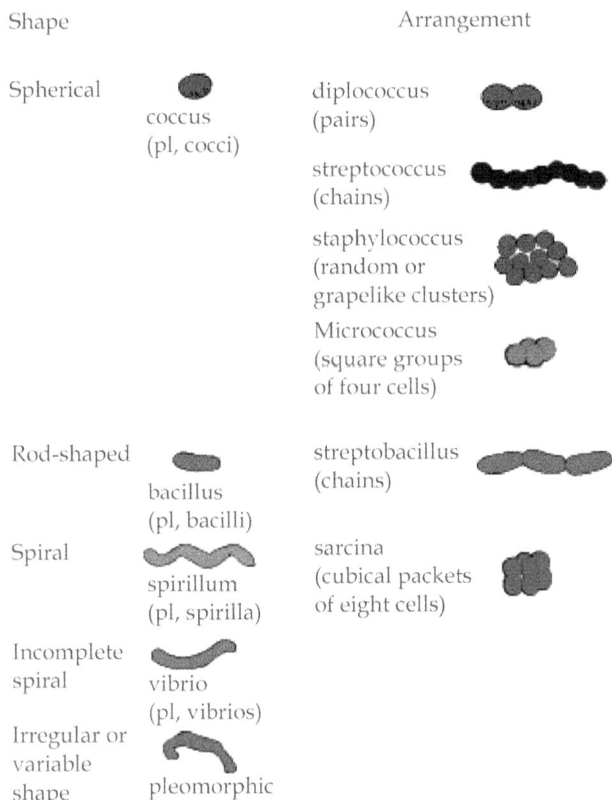

Fig. 9.2 Common bacterial shape.

Observation

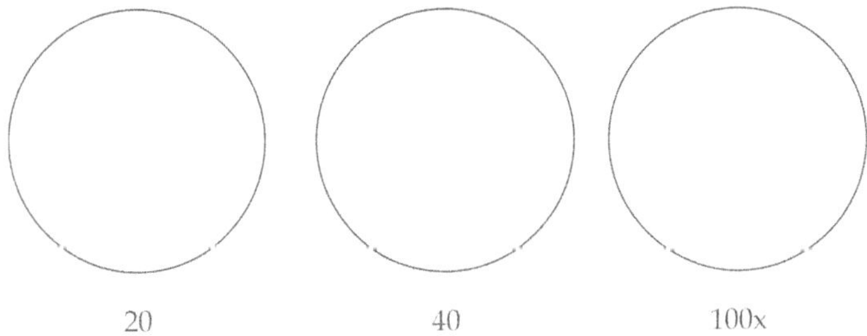

Observation

S. No.	Characterization	Observation
1	Color	
2	Shape	
3	Size	
4	Arrangement	

Report

Chapter 10

Gram Staining

Object

1. To understand the principle of Gram stain.

2. To perform the Gram staining.

Principle

The most important differential stain used in bacteriology is the gram stain, named after Dr. Christian Gram. It divides bacterial cells into two major groups, gram positive and gram negative, which makes it essential tool for classification and differentiation of microorganisms.

1. *Gram-positive bacteria:* After staining a bacteria with crystal violet, if its cell wall resists decolourisation by washing with a decolourising agent (ethanol or acetone), it is a gram-positive bacteria. Examples: Bacillus, Staphylococcus.

2. *Gram-negative bacteria:* After staining a bacteria with crystal violet, if its cell wall allows to undergo decolourisation by washing with a decolourising agent (ethanol or acetone), it is a gram-negative bacteria. Examples: *Escherichia, Salmonella, Vibrio.*

Differentiation of bacteria into gram-positive and gram-negative groups provides the most important clue for proceeding further in proper direction for identification of unknown bacteria. It is also useful for simple differentiation of bacteria into gram-positive and gram-negative groups. It also gives an idea about the shape and arrangement of the bacteria cells.

The differential staining technique requires at least three chemical reagents which are applied subsequently to a heat fixed smear. The first reagent is called the primary stain which imparts its color to all the cells. In order to establish a color contrast, a decolorizing agent is used based up on the chemical composition of cellular components; it may or may not remove the primary stain from the entire cell or only from certain cell structures. The final reagent is the counter stain, has a contrasting color to that of the primary stain. Following decolorizing, if the primary stain is not washed out, the counter stain cannot be absorbed and the cell or its components will retain the color of the primary stain. If the primary stain is removed, the decolorized cellular components will accept and assume the contrasting color of the counter stain. In this way, cell types or their structures can be distinguished from each other on the basis of the stain that is retained.

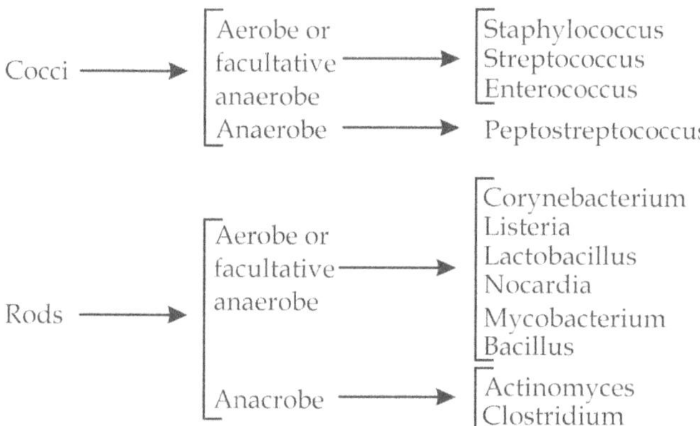

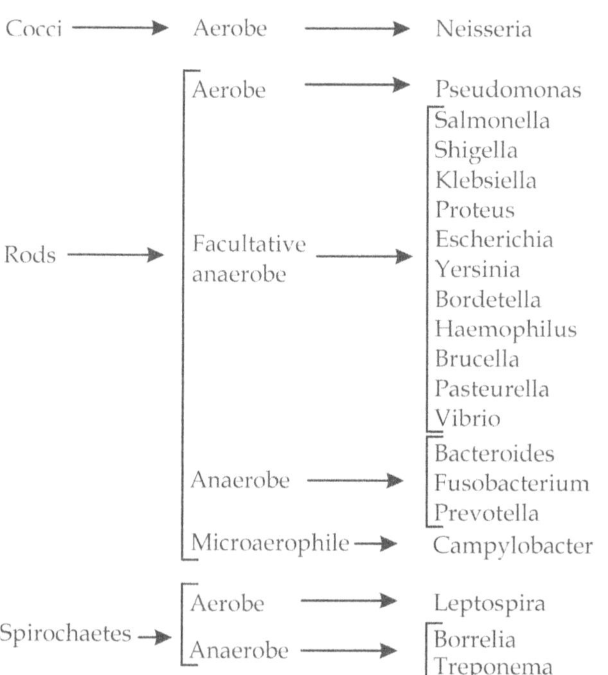

Fig. 10.1 Gram positive & gram negative bacteria.

The gram stain uses four different reagents.

Primary stain: Crystal violet – this violet stain is used first and stains all cells purple.

Mordant: Gram's Iodine – this reagent serves as mordant, a substance that forms an insoluble complex by binding to the primary stain. The resultant crystal violet – Iodine complex (CV-I) serves to intensify the color of the stain, and all the cells will appear purple black at this point. In grams positive cells only, this CV-I complex binds to the magnesium – ribonucleic acid component of the cell wall. The resultant Magnesium –ribonucleic acid –crystal violet – iodine complex (Mg-RNA-CV-I) is more difficult to remove than the smaller CV- I complex.

Decolorizing agent: Ethyl Alcohol, 95% - this reagent serves a dual function as a lipid solvent and as protein dehydrating agent. Its action is determined by the lipid concentration of the microbial cell wall. In gram positive cells, the low lipid concentration is important to retention of the Mg-RNA-CV-I complex. Therefore, the small amount of lipid content is readily dissolved by the action of the alcohol, causing formation of minute cell wall pores. These are then closed by alcohol's dehydrating effect. As a consequence, the tightly bound primary stain is difficult to remove, and the cells remain purple.

In gram negative cells, the high lipid concentration found in outer layers of the cell wall is dissolved by the alcohol, creating large pores in the cell wall that do not close appreciably on dehydration of cell wall proteins. This facilitates release of the unbound CV-I complex living these cells colorless or unstained.

Counter stain: Safranin – this is the final reagent, used to stain red those cells that have been previously decolorized. Since only gram-negative cells undergo decolonization, they may now absorb the counter stain. Gram positive cells retain the purple color of the primary stain.

Material Required

Instrument required: Clean microscope slides, bibulous paper, inoculating loop and needle, sterile distilled water, methylene blue, crystal violet (1% aqueous solution), Grams iodine, 95% ethyl alcohol, and Safranin. Bunsen burner, slide rack, Microscope, immersion oil, lens paper and lens cleaner.

Culture: 24- to 48-hr broth or agar slants of *E. coli* and *Bacillus subtillis.*

Procedure: (Illustration shown in the diagram)

1. A slide is cleaned properly under tap water, such that water does not remain as drops on its surface. The adhering water is wiped out with bibulous paper and the slide is air-dried.

2. A smear of bacteria is prepared at the center of the slide in two methods as follows.

    (a) If a bacterium grown on agar plate or agar slant is to be observed, a drop of water is put at the center of the slide and a loop of bacteria from the plate or slant is transferred to it by a loop sterilized over flame. Then, by slow rotation of the loop in the drop, a bacteria suspension is made and it is spread till a smear is obtained.

    (b) If a bacterium grown in liquid broth is to be observed, a drop of the bacteria suspension is directly placed at the center of the slide by a flame-sterilized loop and a smear is made by spreading.

3. The smear is air-dried.

4. The smear is fixed by heating. Heating results in coagulation of the cellular proteins, due to which the cells stick to the slide surface and do not get washed away during staining, Heat- fixation is done by quickly passing the slide high above a flame 2-3 times, with the smear surface facing upward, so that the smear does not get heated up.

5. The slide is kept on a staining tray and flooded with the primary stain, crystal violet, for 1 minute.

6. Excess stain is washed away from the smear under gently-flowing tap water, in such a way that, water does not fall directly on the smear.

7. The smear is flooded with the mordant, gram's iodine, for 1 minute.

8. Excess mordant is washed away from the smear under gently-flowing tap water, in such a way that, water does not fall directly on the smear.

9. The smear is flooded with the decolourising agent, 95% ethanol, for 5 seconds, taking care, so that the smear is not over-decolourised.

10. The ethanol is quickly washed away from the smear under gently-flowing tap water, so as to prevent over-decolourisation. Care is taken, so that, water does not fall directly on the smear.

11. The smear is flooded with the counter-stain, safranin, for 1 minute.

12. Excess counter-stain is washed away from the smear under gently-flowing tap water, in such a way that, water does not fall directly on the smear.

13. The slide is blotted dry with bibulous paper.

14. The slide is clipped to the stage of the microscope and the smear observed under low power and high dry objectives.

15. A drop of immersion oil is put on the smear.

16. The smear is observed under oil-immersion objective.

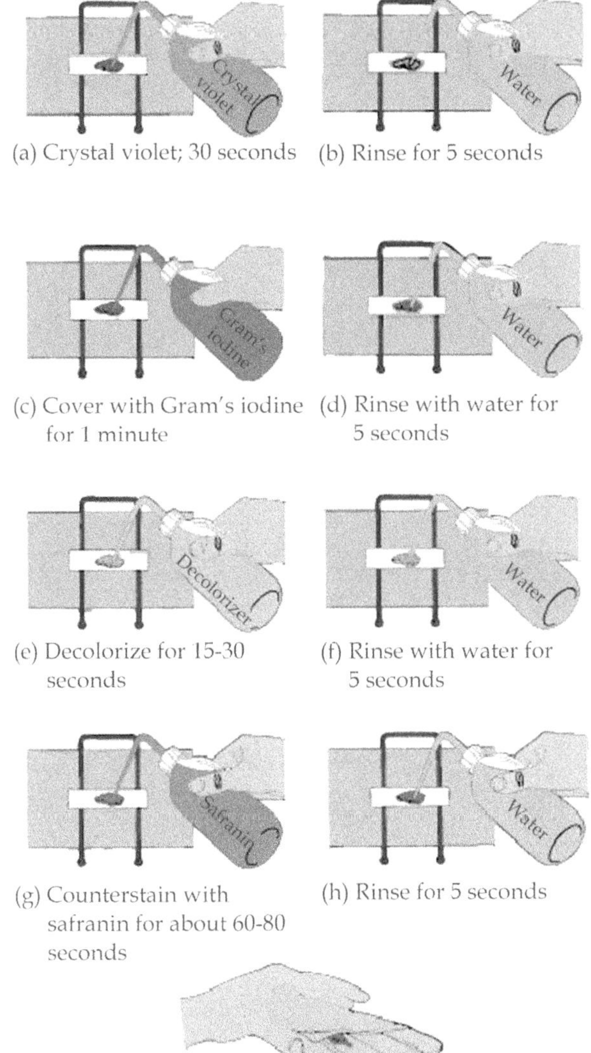

(a) Crystal violet; 30 seconds   (b) Rinse for 5 seconds

(c) Cover with Gram's iodine for 1 minute   (d) Rinse with water for 5 seconds

(e) Decolorize for 15-30 seconds   (f) Rinse with water for 5 seconds

(g) Counterstain with safranin for about 60-80 seconds   (h) Rinse for 5 seconds

Fig. 10.2 Gram stain procedure.

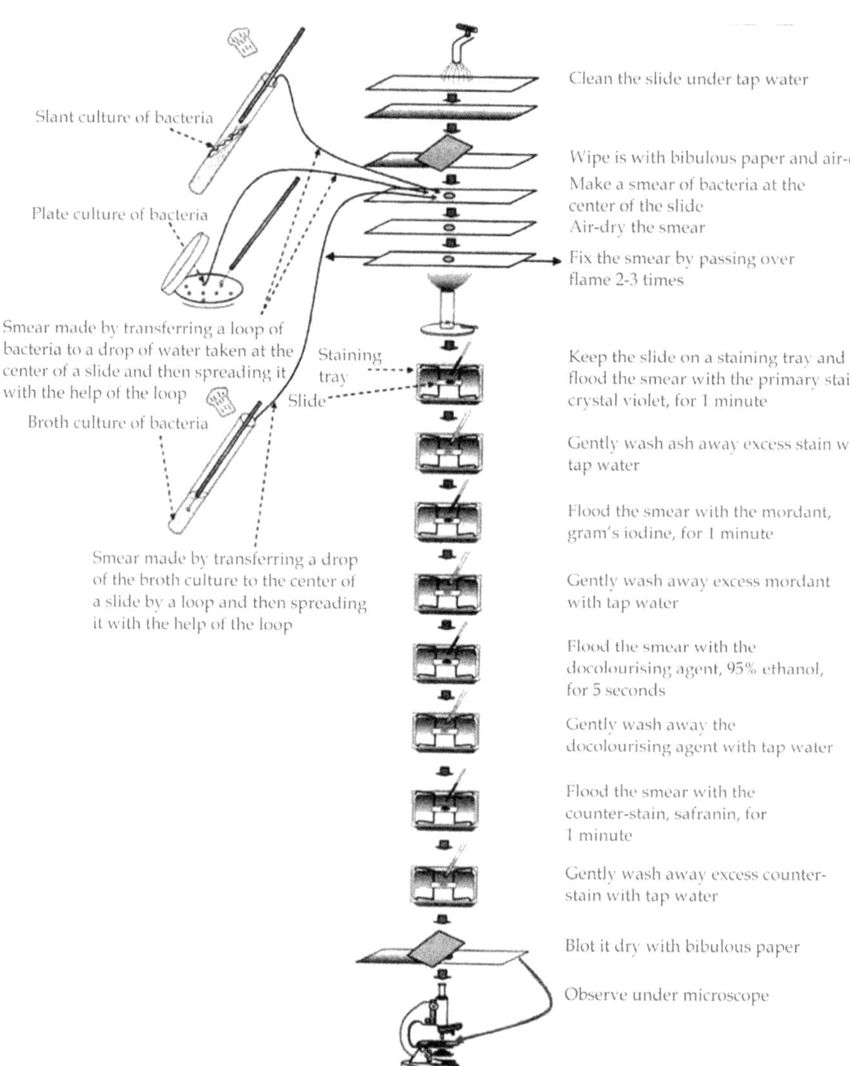

Fig. 10.3 Gram staining of bacteria.

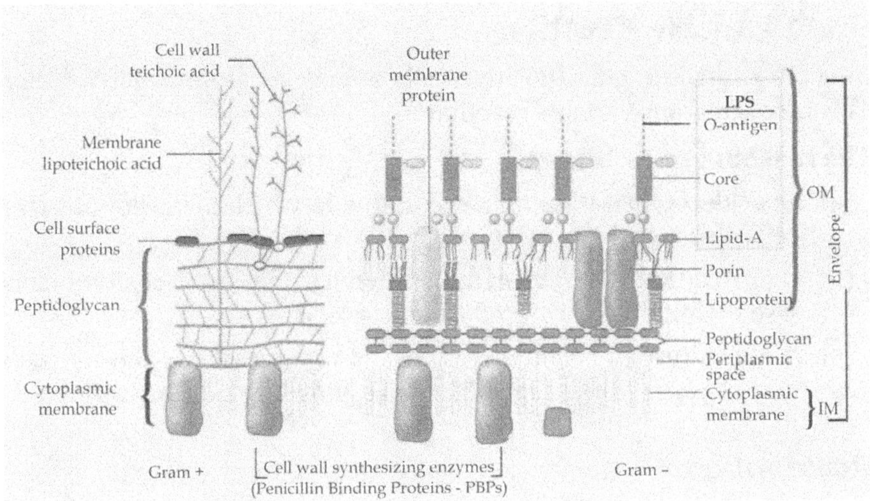

Fig. 10.4 Cell wall of gram positive and gram negative bacteria.

Observations (Under Oil-immersion Objective):

1. **Colour of the cells**

   Purple-blue: Gram-positive bacteria

   Pink-red: Gram-negative bacteria

2. **Shape of bacteria**

   Spherical (coccus)

   Rod-shaped (bacilli)

   Comma-like (vibrio)

   Spiral (spirochetes)

3. **Arrangement of bacteria**

   Pairs (diplobacillus/diplococcus)

   In fours (tetrads)

   In chains (streptococcus/streptobacillus)

   Grape-like clusters (staphylococcus)

   Cuboidal (sarcinae or octet)

4. **Size of bacteria**

   By eye estimation, make drawing of the field under oil-immersion
   objective.

Gram-variable Reaction

In some cases, the gram-positive cells appear as gram-negative cells. This is called gram-variable reaction.

The reasons are as follows

(a) Over-decolourisation may occur, due to which the gram-positive cells also lose their violet colour.

(b) Over-fixation may occur, due to which the gram-positive cells lose their ability to resist decolourisation.

(c) If old culture of bacteria is used, the components of the cell wall may change with the age of the cells allowing decolourisation.

Observation

S. No.	Characterization	Observation
1	Color	
2	Shape	
3	Size	
4	Arrangement	
5	Gram reaction	

Report

Chapter 11

Negative Staining

Object

1. To understand the principle of Negative staining.
2. To perform the Negative staining.

Principles

Sometimes the use of harsh staining procedures or heat-fixing techniques can alter the morphological characteristics of the cells. In some cases the bacterium does not stain well (e.g., some of the spirochetes). The Negative staining is convenient to determine overall bacterial morphology and also good for viewing capsules.

Negative, indirect, or **background staining** is achieved by mixing bacteria with an acidic stain such as nigrosin, India ink, or eosin, and then spreading out the mixture on a slide to form a film. This stain will not penetrate and stain the bacterial cells due to repulsion between the negative charge of the stains and the negatively charged bacterial wall. Instead, these stains either produce a deposit around the bacteria or produce a dark background so that the bacteria appear as unstained cells with a clear area around them.

Material Required

Instrument required: Clean microscope slides, bibulous paper, inoculating loop and needle, sterile distilled water, Dorner's nigrosin solution, India ink, or eosin blue Bunsen burner, slide rack, microscope, immersion oil, lens paper and lens cleaner.

Culture: 24- to 48-hr broth or agar slants of *E. coli* and *Bacillus subtillis.*

Procedure (illustration show in the diagram)

1. With a glassware marking pen, label the left-hand corner of glass slides with the names of the respective bacteria.

2. With the help of an inoculating loop, place a drop of bacteria at one end of a clean glass slide.

3. Then add 1 to 2 drop of nigrosin, India ink, or eosin solution to the bacteria and mix thoroughly.

4. Spread the mixture over the slide using another slide, which is inclined at a 45° angle so that the bacteria-nigrosin solution spreads across its edge. The slide is then pushed across the surface of the first slide in order to form a smear that is thick at one end and thin at the other. This is known as a **thin smear.**

5. Allow the smear to air dry.

6. Observe the slide under the microscope.

7. Record the reading.

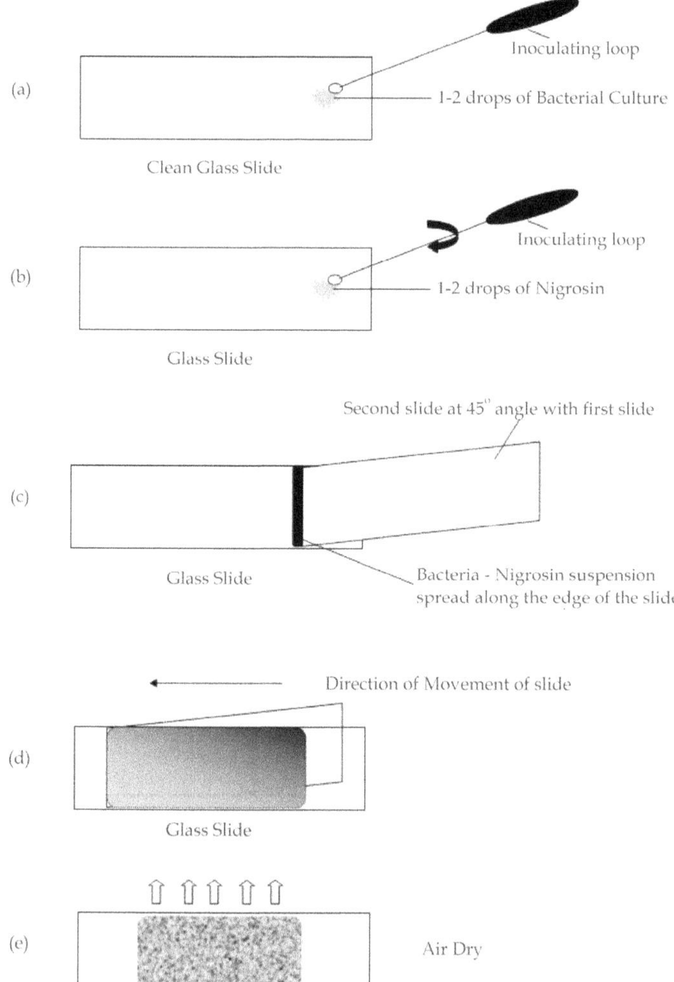

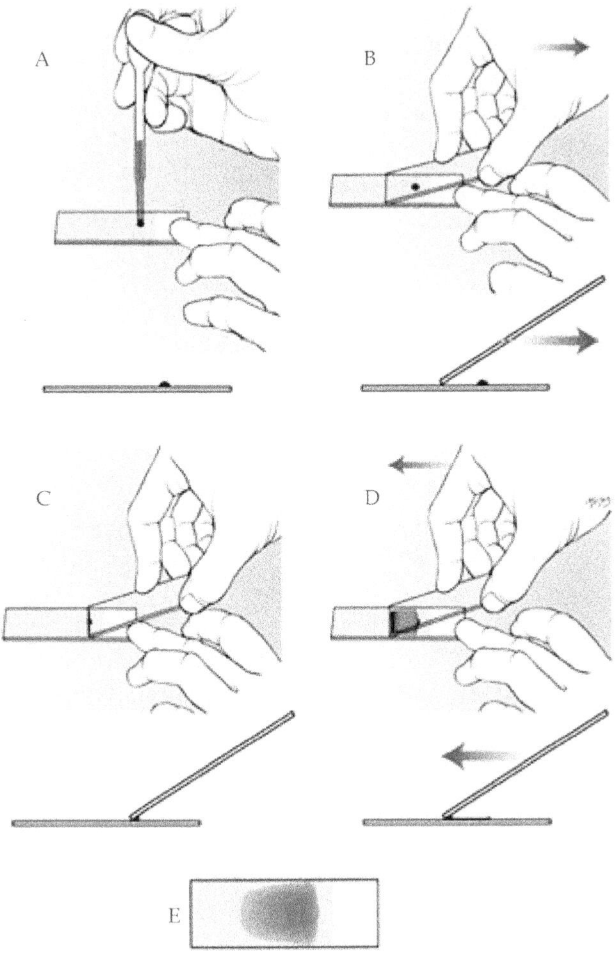

Fig. 11.1 Negative staining procedure and thin smear preparation.

Observation

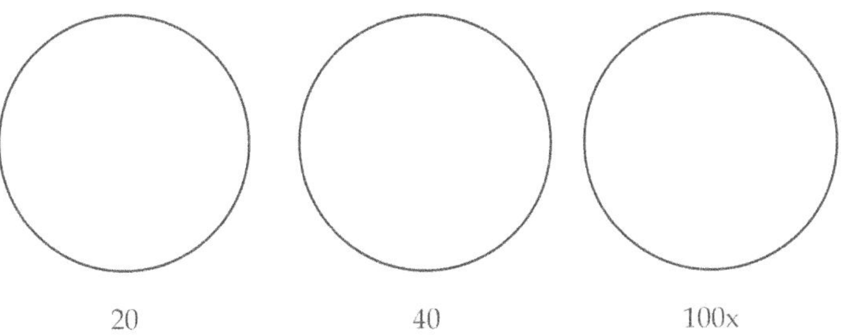

Observation

S. No.	Characterization	Observation
1	Shape	
2	Size	
3	Arrangement	

Report

Chapter 12

Acid Fast Staining – Ziehl-Neelsen Staining

Object

1. To understand the basic principle of acid fast staining.
2. To perform the Acid Fast Staining.

Principle

The Ziehl–Neelsen stain, also known as the acid-fast stain, was first described by the bacteriologist Franz Ziehl (1859–1926) and the pathologist Friedrich Neelsen (1854–1898). It is a special bacteriological stain used to identify acid-fast organisms, mainly Mycobacterium. *Mycobacterium tuberculosis, Mycobacterium leprae, Mycobacterium kansasii, Mycobacterium marinum,* and members of the *Mycobacterium avium* complex.

The mycobacterium has a special contain large amounts of lipid substances within their cell walls called mycolic acid, which resist staining by ordinary methods such as a Gram stain. The presence of the mycolic acid produces a characteristic thick waxy layer around the cell wall which is extremely difficult for the stain to penetrate and once the stain is penetrated it cannot be readily removed also. In the acid fast staining technique three different staining agents are used.

1. ***Primary Stain:*** Carbol fuchsin: It is a dark red stain in 5% phenol, which is soluble in lipoidal cell wall of the mycobacterium, it penetrate the bacterium & retained. The penetration can be enhanced by applying the heat. The primary stain will impart red color to the cell.

2. ***Decolorizing agent:*** Acid-Alcohol (3%HCl + 95% Ethanol): Prior to the application of decolorizing agent the smear is cooled,

which allows the waxy cell layer get hardened. On application of the decolorizing agent the acid fast stain will be resistant to decolonization process because of the wax cell wall; where as the non acid fast bacteria will get decolorized because of the absence of waxy layer.

3. ***Counter Stain:*** Methylene Blue: This will impart blue color to the non acid fast bacteria because it had got decolorized in the previous step, so we will get an contrast color.

Material Required

Instrument required: Clean microscope slides, bibulous paper, inoculating loop and needle, sterile distilled water, Carbol fuchsin, acid-alcohol, Methylene Blue Bunsen burner, slide rack, Microscope, immersion oil, lens paper and lens cleaner.

Culture: 96 hr trypticase soy broth culture of E. *coli* and *Mycobacterium smegmatis.*

Procedure (illustration show in the diagram)

1. With a glassware marking pen, label the left-hand corner of glass slides with the names of the respective bacteria.
2. Prepare the smear as discussed earlier.
3. Flood the smear with Carbol fuchsin place over the beaker containing boiling water and allow the preparation to steam for 5 minutes. (don't allow the stain to evaporate, add stain as needed)
4. Cool the slide and wash with running tap water.
5. Decolorize by adding acid-alcohol drop wise until the alcohol run clears or thin red color.
6. Wash with running tap water immediately.
7. Counter stain with methylene blue for 2 minutes and wash with running tap water.
8. Allow the smear to air dry.
9. Observe the slide under the microscope under oil immersion.
10. Record the reading.

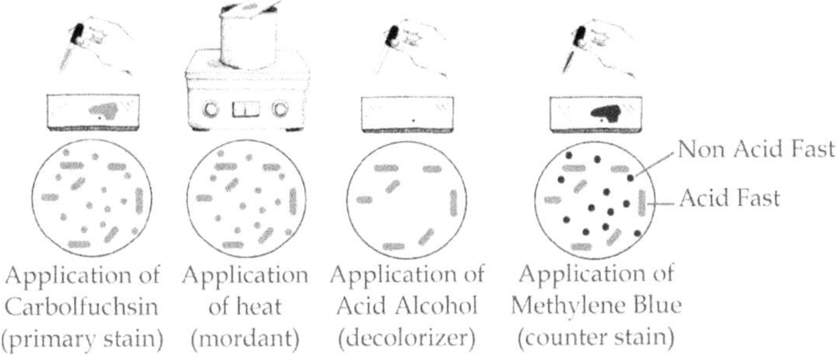

Fig. 12.1 Acid fast staining - Ziehl–Neelsen staining.

Observation

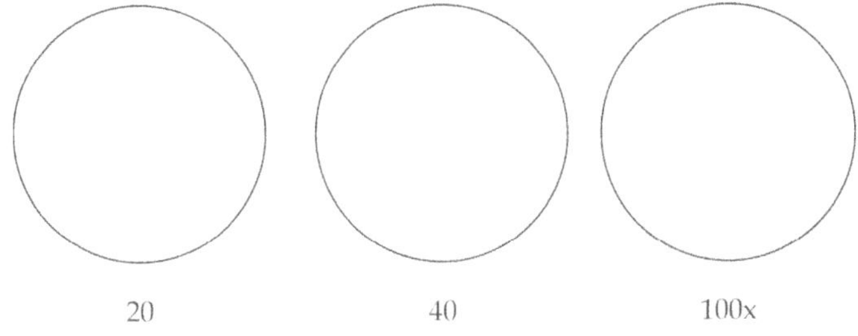

Observation

S. No.	Characterization	Observation
1	Shape	
2	Size	
3	Arrangement	
4	Cell color	
5	Acid fast reaction	

Report

Chapter 13

Spore Staining

Object

1. To understand the basic principle of spore staining technique (Schaeffer–Fulton mehod).
2. To perform the spore staining.

Principle

The Schaeffer–Fulton stain is a technique designed to isolate endospores from vegetative cells by staining. The bacteria belong to *Clostridium* and *Bacillius* species can exists metabolically active vegetative cell or inactive highly resistant spores. Under the unfavorable environmental condition the vegetative cell undergo sporogenesis and from endospores and if the unfavorable condition persists it get released as spores. The spores are highly resistant to heat, radiation, desiccation and chemical agents. When the favorable condition returns the spores undergoes germination process and forms vegetative cells.

The spore staining done by three different agents

1. ***Primary stain – Malachite Green:*** The primary stain will impart stain both the vegetative cells and spores, since the spore are resistant to chemical agents the penetration of primary stain can be enhanced by applying the heat.
2. ***Decolorizing agent – Water:*** Once spore get stained with the primary staining agent, it is very difficult to decolorize with water, where as the vegetative cell gets decolorized easily.
3. ***Counter Stain – Safranin:*** The contrast red color dye is used to stain the decolorized vegetative cells.

Material Required

Instrument required: Clean microscope slides, bibulous paper, inoculating loop and needle, sterile distilled water, Malachite Green,

Safranin, Bunsen burner, slide rack, Microscope, immersion oil, lens paper and lens cleaner.

Culture: 48 to 72 hr Thioglycolate culture of *Clostridium butyricum.*

Procedure (illustration show in the diagram)

1. With a glassware marking pen, label the left-hand corner of glass slides with the names of the respective bacteria.

2. Prepare the smear as discussed earlier.

3. Flood the smear with Malachite Green place over the beaker containing boiling water and allow the preparation to steam for 2 to 3 minutes. (don't allow the stain to evaporate, add stain as needed and also prevent the stain from boiling)

4. Cool the slide and wash with running tap water.

5. Counter stain with Safranin for 30 seconds and wash with running tap water.

6. Allow the smear to air dry.

7. Observe the slide under the microscope under oil immersion.

8. Record the reading.

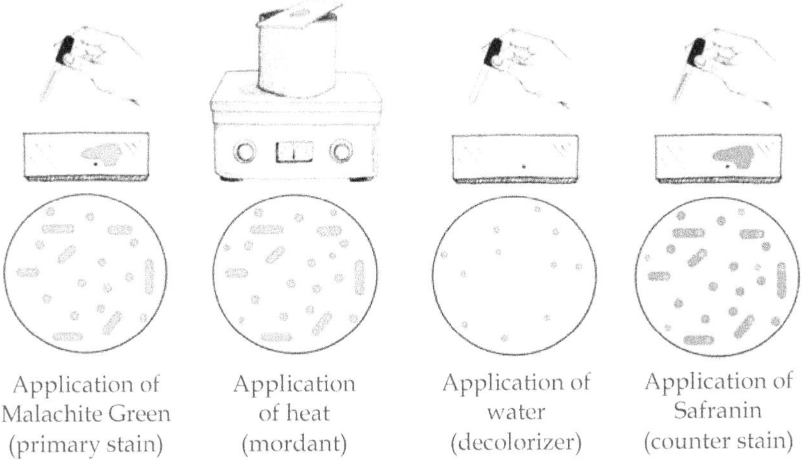

Fig. 13.1 Spore staining.

Observation

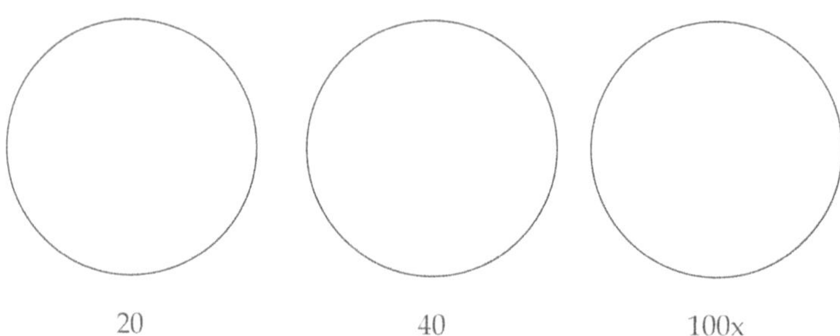

Observation

S. No.	Characterization	Observation
1	Color of Spores	
2	Color of Vegetative cells	
3	Location of Endspores	

Report

Chapter 14

Capsule Staining

Object

1. To understand the basic principle of Capsule staining technique (Anthony method).
2. To perform the Capsule Staining.

Principle

Capsule is the gelatinous outer layer formed by the secretion of the bacteria outside the cell wall. The bacteria which contain the capsule are virulent because it inhibits the penetration of antibiotic through the cell wall. The capsule is made up of glycol protein, polysaccharide or a poly peptide.

The capsule stains with two agents:

1. ***Primary Stain: Crystal violet (1% aqueous):*** A violet stain is applied on not heat fixed smear.
2. ***Decolorizing agent – Copper sulfate (20%):*** The copper sulfate is used as decolorizing agent instead of water because water can easily dissolve the capsule and copper sulfate washes the purple primary stain of the capsule only without affecting the cell. The decolorized capsule will take the copper sulfate and appears blue in contrast to deep purple color of the cell.

Material Required

Instrument required: Clean microscope slides, bibulous paper, inoculating loop and needle, sterile distilled water, 1% crystal violet, 20% copper sulfate, Bunsen burner, slide rack, Microscope, immersion oil, lens paper and lens cleaner.

Culture: 48 hr skimmed milk culture of *Leuconostoc mesenteroides* and *Enterobacter aerogenes.*

Procedure (illustration show in the diagram)

1. With a glassware marking pen, label the left-hand corner of glass slides with the names of the respective bacteria.

2. Place some drops of crystal violet at the center of slide and add loop full of microorganism aseptically and with the help of another slide spread to form a thin smear. Stand for 5 to 7 minutes.

3. Allow the smear to air dry.

4. Wash smear with 20% copper sulfate solution, gently blot dry it.

5. Observe the slide under the microscope in oil immersion.

6. Record the reading.

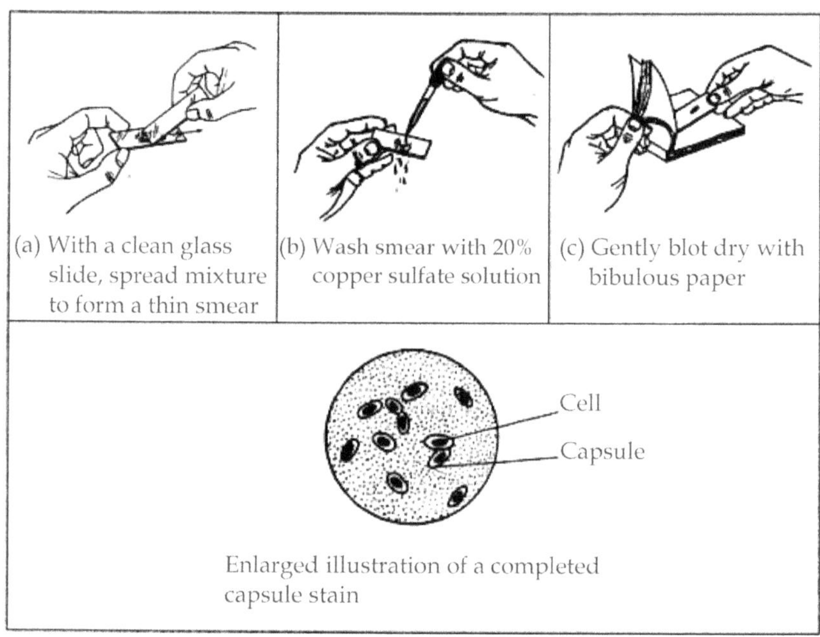

Fig. 14.1 Capsule Staining.

Observation

20X	40X	100 X (oil)

Observation

S. No.	Characterization	Observation
1	Color of Capsule	
2	Color of Vegetative cells	
3	Size of Capsule	

Report

Chapter 15

Motility of Bacteria (Hanging Drop Method)

Object

1. To perform the hanging drop procedure for microscopic examination of motility of bacteria.

Principle

Because of their small size Bacteria and refractive index becomes difficult to observe readily under microscopic without staining. Examination of living microorganisms is useful to

1. Observe cell activities such as motility and binary fission.

2. Observe the natural sizes and shapes of the cells, since heat fixation and exposure to chemicals during staining causes some degree of distortion.

Two general techniques are used for observing the live bacterial preparations. They are:

1. Wet mount technique: the organisms are suspended in a liquid spread on the slide and observed.

2. Hanging drop method: this method is used to observe the motility of the organism using a cavity slide.

Motile strains of bacteria posses filamentous appendages known as flagella, which effect screw like propulsive movements and act as organelles of locomotion. A flagellum is a long, thin filament, twisted spirally. It is about 0.02µm thick and is usually several times the length of bacterial cell. According to the species there may be one or several flagella. The flagella are made up of a protein called flagellin.

A microbial suspension is placed on the cover slip. The slide with a concave depression lined with petroleum jelly is inverted over the drop to produce a hanging drop of the preparation.

On microscopic observation the bacteria can be seen swimming in different directions across the field with a darting, wriggling or tumbling movement. True motility may be distinguished from the Brownian movement, which is a rapid oscillation of each bacterium within a very limited area due to the bombardment by the water molecule.

Material Required

Instrument required: Clean Concave depression slides, Cover slip, bibulous paper, inoculating loop and needle, sterile distilled water, petroleum jelly, Bunsen burner, slide rack, Microscope, immersion oil, lens paper and lens cleaner.

Culture: 24 hour cultures of *Escherichia coli* and *Bacillus subtillis.*

Procedure

1. A ring of petroleum jelly was applied around the concavity of the depression slide.

2. Using sterile technique, a loopful of culture was placed in the centre of the clean cover slip.

3. The depression slide was placed with the concave surface facing down, over the cover slip so that the depression covers the drop of culture. The slide was pressed gently to form a seal between the slide and cover slip.

4. The slide was turned right side up so that the drop continues to adhere to the inner surface of the cover slip.

5. The drop of culture was first focused under the low power objective with reduced light. Then a drop of oil was placed over the cover slip and observed under oil immersion for the detailed observation.

(a)

Tooth Pick
Slide concavity
Vaseline ring
Clean Glass Slide

(b)

Inoculating loop
Bacterial Culture
Cover slip

(c)

Move slide to Cover slip
Drops of Bacterial Culture

(d)

Turn Slide Over

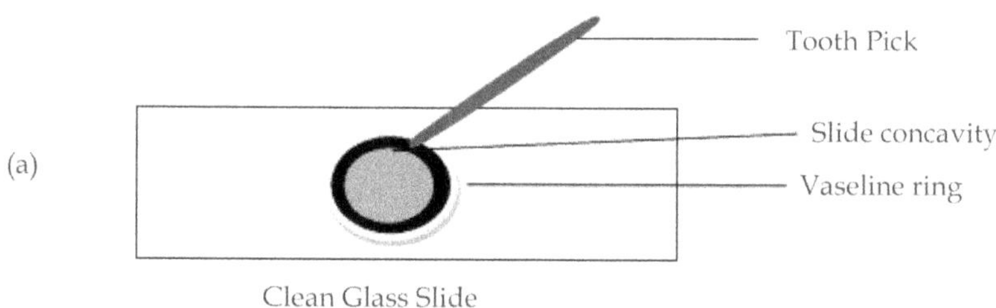

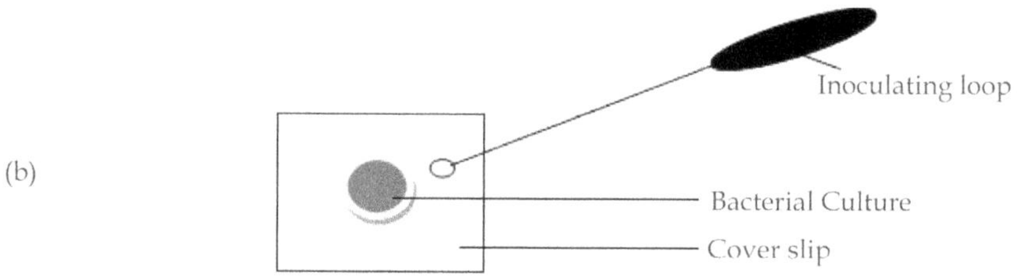

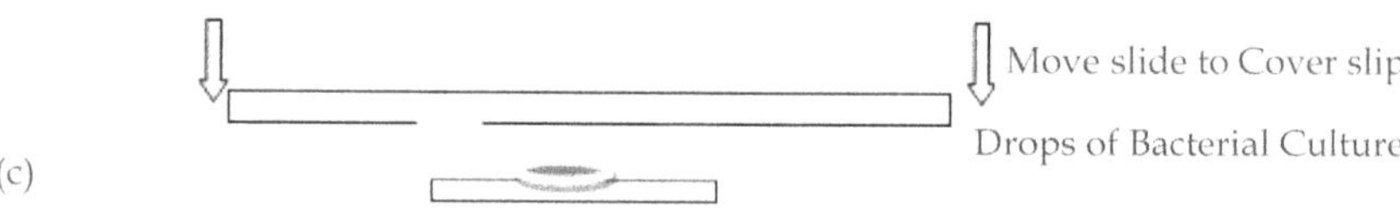

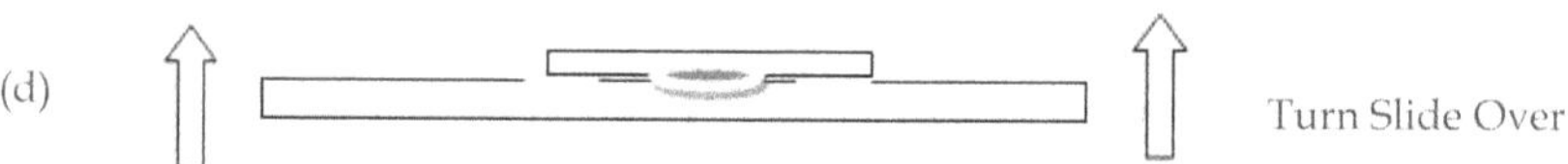

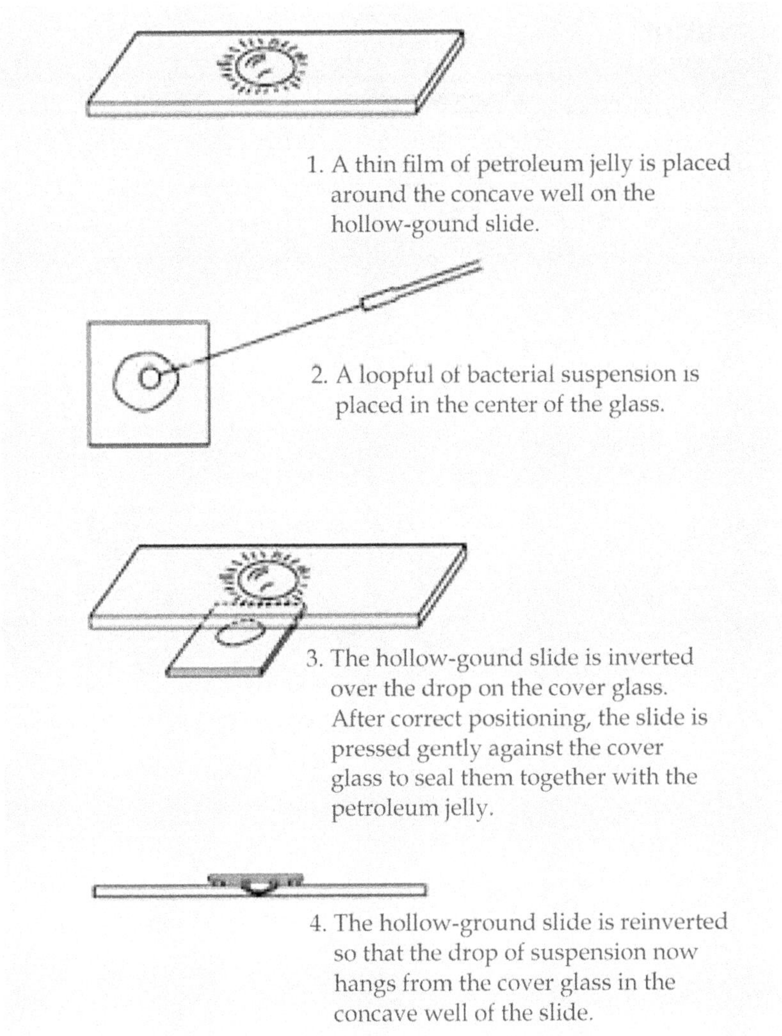

1. A thin film of petroleum jelly is placed around the concave well on the hollow-gound slide.

2. A loopful of bacterial suspension is placed in the center of the glass.

3. The hollow-gound slide is inverted over the drop on the cover glass. After correct positioning, the slide is pressed gently against the cover glass to seal them together with the petroleum jelly.

4. The hollow-ground slide is reinverted so that the drop of suspension now hangs from the cover glass in the concave well of the slide.

Fig. 15.1 Preparation of hanging drop slide.

Observation

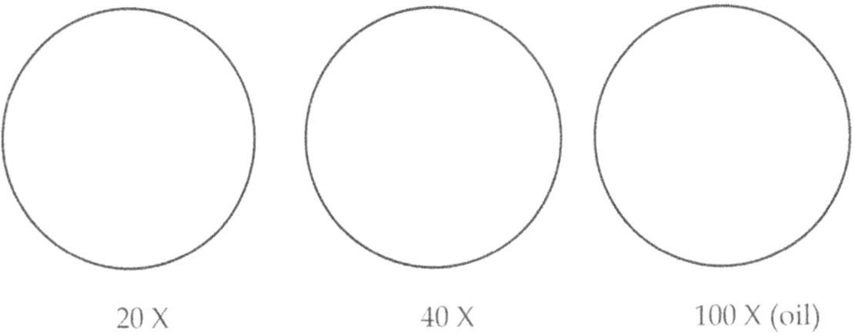

20 X   40 X   100 X (oil)

Observation

S. No.	Characterization	Observation
1	Motility of bacteria	
2	Shape of bacteria	
3	Size of bacteria	
4	Arrangement of Bacteria	

Report

PART - IV

BIOCHEMICAL CHARACTERIZATION OF BACTERIA

Chapter 16

Acetamide Utilization Test

Object

1. To understand the biochemical basis of Acetamide Utilization Test.
2. To perform Acetamide Utilization Test.

Principle

This test is performed for differentiating the *pseudomonas aeruginosa* from other non glucose fermenting gram negative rod shaped bacteria.

It is performed to test the bacteria that have the ability to acetamide as sole carbon source and inorganic ammonium salts as sole nitrogen source. The bacteria which give the positive results to the test have the ability to metabolize acetamide to ammonia by the enzymatic action of acylamidase. The formation of ammonia shifts the pH of the medium to alkaline region, which can be identified by the change in color of the media from green to blue by the indicator present in the medium bromthymol blue.

Material Required

Culture: 24 hour cultures of pseudomonas aeruginosa.

Medium: Acetamide Utilization Medium.

Table 16.1

S. No.	Composition	Amount for 1000 mL
1	Sodium Chloride	5.0 gm
2	Magnesium Sulfate	0.2 gm
3	Ammonium Phosphate monobasic	1.0 gm
4	Potassium phosphate dibasic	1.0 gm
5	Acetamide	10.0 gm
6	Agar	15.0 gm
7	Bromthymol Blue	0.08 gm
8	Distill Water	1000 mL
pH – 6.8, Store at 2-8 ºC		

Instrument required: Inoculating loop and needle, sterile distilled water, Laminar airflow cabinet and Incubator.

Procedure

1. Inoculate the microorganism by means of streaking the Acetamide Utilization Medium slant back and forth aseptically.
2. Plug with cotton and incubate at 35 to 37°C for 4 days.
3. Observe the color change from green to blue of the slant.

Observation

S. No	Characterization	Observation
1	Color of the slant	
2	Acetamide Utilization	

Report

Chapter 17

Acetate Utilization Test

Object

1. To understand the biochemical basis of Acetate Utilization Test.
2. To perform Acetate Utilization Test.

Principle

This test is performed for differentiating the *Shigella sp.* from *Escherichia coli* because 80% of the *E. coli* strains utilize acetate, whereas the *shigella* species is incapable of utilization of acetate.

It is performed to test the bacteria that have the ability to utilize acetate as sole carbon source and inorganic ammonium as sole nitrogen source. The bacteria which give the positive results to the test have the ability to metabolize acetate, ammonium salts into ammonia, which shifts the pH of the medium to alkaline region. The shift of pH turns the bromothymol blue indicator in the medium from green to blue.

Material Required

Culture: 24 hour cultures of *Shigella* sp. and *Escherichia coli.*

Medium: Acetate Utilization Medium.

Table 17.1

S. No.	Composition	Amount for 1000 mL
1	Sodium Chloride	5.0 gm
2	Magnesium Sulfate	0.1 gm
3	Ammonium Phosphate monobasic	1.0 gm
4	Potassium phosphate dibasic	1.0 gm
5	Sodium acetate	2.0 gm
6	Agar	20.0 gm
7	Bromthymol Blue	0.08 gm
8	Distill Water	1000 mL
pH – 6.7		

Media required: 3 sodium acetate agar slants.

Instrument required: Inoculating loop and needle, sterile distilled water, laminar airflow cabinet and Incubator.

Procedure

1. Inoculate the microorganism *Shigella sp.* and *Escherichia coli* by means of streaking the appropriately marked sodium acetate agar slants back and forth aseptically.
2. Plug with cotton and incubate at 35 to 37ºC for 5 days.
3. Observe the color change from green to blue of the slant.

Observation

S. No.	Characterization	Observation
1	Color of the slant	
2	Acetate Utilization	

Report

Chapter 18

AL (δ-Amino Levelunic Acid) Test for Porphyrin Synthesis

Object

1. To understand the biochemical basis of ALA – Test for Porphyrin Synthesis.
2. To perform ALA – Test for Porphyrin Synthesis.

Principle

This test is performed for determining the growth requirement for hemin (X-factor) in the identification of *Haemophilus sp.*

It is performed to test the organisms which do not require hemin for growth can produce porphobilinogen from ALA by the activation of the enzyme porphobilinogen synthase; the porphobilinogen is converted to protoporphyrin IV (the precursor of hemin).

The presence of porphyrin is detected by emission of flouresence under UV light (360nm) in red orange color.

If no flouresence is detected then the test tube is treated with indole to test the presence of porphobilinogen, which is also consider as positive result (Presence of porphobilinogen synthase).

Material Required

Culture

24hour cultures of *Haemophilius influenza* (negative control – no red flouresence), *Haemophilius parainfluenza* (positive control –red flouresence) and test organism.

Chemical Required

1. 33.5mg of ALA
2. 19.72 mg of $MgSO_4.7H_2O$

3. 0.1M Sorensen's phosphate buffer, pH – 6.9

4. Kovacs indole reagent

Preparation of 0.1M Sorensen's Phosphate Buffer, pH – 6.9

1. 3.15 gm of $NaH_2PO_4.H_2O$ and 7.4 gm of $Na_2HPO_4.H_2O$ is dissolved in 500ml of deionized water.

2. The pH was adjusted with either 0.1M HCl or 0.1M NaOH

Preparation of ALA Reagent

1. 33.5 mg of ALA and 19.72 mg of MgSO4.7H2O is dissolved in 100ml of 0.1M Sorensen's phosphate buffer, pH – 6.9

Instrument Required

Filter paper, test tubes, petri dish, Inoculating loop, UV light, laminar airflow cabinet and Incubator.

Procedure 1: Filter Paper Method

1. Place a sterile filter paper fit to the sterilized Petri dish

2. Mark the filter paper with circle of 10mm in diameter for test. Positive and negative control

3. Inoculate the center of the mark with colony of test, positive and negative microorganism.

4. Slowly pour thawed ALA reagent over filter paper. Covering the Petri dish.

5. Incubate at 35 °C for 2hrs in a non – CO_2 incubator.

6. Observe the reaction in UV light for fluorescence in a dark room.

7. If positive control also doesn't shown fluorescence, than reincubate for another 2 to 4 hrs.

Procedure 2: Tube Method

1. Inoculate each test tube containing 0.5ml of ALA reagent with microorganism.

2. Incubate at 35 °C for 2hrs in a non – CO_2 incubator.

3. Observe the reaction in UV light for fluorescence in a dark room.

4. If positive control also doesn't shown fluorescence, than reincubate for another 2 to 4 hrs.

Observation

S. No.	Characterization	Observation
1	Color of the fluorescence	
2	Porphyrin Synthesis	

Report

Chapter 19

Carbohydrate Utilization Test

Object

1. To understand the biochemical basis of Carbohydrate Utilization Test.
2. To perform Carbohydrate Utilization Test.

Principle

This test is performed to check the ability of the microorganism to utilize carbohydrate. The media used for this test contains 1% carbohydrate and pH indicator and a protein source. 1% concentration of carbohydrate is optimal for most reactions and there is no possibility of reversal reactions. This test is will also differentiate the organism based on the type of indicator used and color produced, which are shown in the Table 19.1.

Table 19.1

S. No.	Type of indicator used in media	Color change	Type of organism
1	Bromcresol purple	Purple to yellow at pH 5.2	Gram positive
2	Andrade's indicator- acid fuchsin	Straw to fuchsin red, when pH reduced (acid production)	Gram negative - rod
3	Neutral red or phenol red	Red to yellow with drop in pH (acid production)	Gram negative - rod

Bacteria can be divided by their ability to degrade carbohydrate aerobically or anaerobically. The anaerobic fermentation can at the bottom of the tube and aerobic oxidation can be observed at the top of the tube. The bacterium is performing the anaerobic fermentation or aerobic oxidation can be identified by **Triple sugar iron test** or **Klingers iron agar.**

If the bacteria undergoes fermentation is identified by yellow butt formation, if it is not than the microorganism is oxidizer and non utilizer. Organism is determined to be non-glucose fermentating **Oxidative Fermentation** is done to determine the organism is not producing acid from glucose by fermentation, this can be determined by adding bromthymol blue, which turns yellow when acid is produced from glucose. Similarly it is carried out for non glucose or alternative carbohydrate fermenting bacteria also.

The **Cystine Trypticase Agar test** is done to determine the bacteria which are too fastidious for growth. The conversion of carbohydrate to acid is identified by the phenol red indicator, which turns from red to yellow when the pH is 6.8. The microorganism which gives positive reaction includes *Neisseria, Haemophilius, Kingella, Capnocytophaga, Actinobacillus* and lopid requiring gram positive rods.

The production of gas from fermentation of sugars by two methods

1. The microorganism is inoculated in agar tubes and the disruption of agar is the evident of gas production.

2. Durham tube is inverted and placed inside the broth medium inoculated with microorganism, the entrapment of gas in the durham's tube is visually observed for the production of gas.

3. The hot loop method is used for determining fastidious gram negative rods; a red hot loop is near the side of the test tube containing the 48hr to 72hr culture of microorganism, gas bubble is released along with the tube.

Test 1: Purple Broth Test

Material Required

Media composition of Purple broth

Table 19.2

S. No.	Composition	Amount
1	Peptone	10.00 gm
2	Sodium chloride	5.00 gm
3	Bromcresol purple	0.020 gm
4	Distill water	1000 mL
pH 6.8 ± 0.2		

Media is Sterilize at 121°C for 15 minutes

1% Carbohydrate is filtered and added to the sterilized media.

Culture: 24 hour cultures of *Escherichia coli.*

Instrument Required

Test tube, durham's tube, Inoculating loop, Autoclave, Filtration assembly, Whatman filter paper, laminar airflow cabinet and Incubator.

Procedure

1. The sterilized durham's tube is inverted and placed in the test tube (check for no air is entrapped in the durham's tube)
2. The bacterial culture is inoculated in a sterile purple broth media containing in a test tube aseptically.
3. Incubate for 7 days at 35°C.
4. Observe the results

   (a) If the media turns to yellow color – Acid formation happened pH 5.2 (Positive reaction)
   (b) If the media remains purple color – Alkaline formation happened (Negative reaction)
   (c) Gas production can be identified by bubble production in Durham's tube.

Observation

S. No.	Characterization	Observation
1	Color of the medium	
2	Presence of gas in durham's tube	

Report

Test 2: Cystine Trypticase Agar Test

Media composition of Cystine Trypticase Agar

Table 19.3

S. No.	Composition	Amount
1	Pancreatic digest of casein	20.00 gm
2	Sodium chloride	5.00 gm
3	L-Cystine	0.50 gm
4	Sodium sulphite (Na_2SO_3)	0.50 gm
5	Agar	14.00 gm
6	Phenol red	0.017 gm
7	Distill water	1000 mL
	pH 7.3 ± 0.2	

Media is Sterilize at 121°C for 15minutes

1% Carbohydrate is filtered and added to the sterilized media.

Culture: 24hour cultures of *Neisseria species*

Instrument Required

Test tube, Inoculating loop, Autoclave, Filtration assembly, Whatman filter paper, laminar airflow cabinet and Incubator.

Procedure

1. The bacterial culture is inoculated in a sterile Cystine Trypticase Agar tube aseptically.
2. Inoculate the bacteria in a control tube without carbohydrate for comparison.
3. Incubate for 7 days at 35°C.
4. Observe the results

   (a) If the media turns to yellow color – Acid formation happened pH 6.8 (Positive reaction)

   (b) If the media remains red color or no change with control – Alkaline formation happened (Negative reaction)

Observation

S. No.	Characterization	Observation
1	Color of the medium	

Report

Test 3: Oxidative Fermentation Test

Media composition of Hugh and Leifson's Oxidative Fermentation Basal Medium

S. No.	Composition	Amount
1	Peptone (tryptone)	2.00 gm
2	Sodium chloride	5.00 gm
3	Bromthymol blue	0.03 gm
4	Dipotassium phosphate	0.30 gm
5	Agar	3.00 gm
6	Distill water	1000 ml
	pH 7.1 ± 0.2	

Media is Sterilize at 121°C for 15minutes

Carbohydrate is filtered and added to the sterilized media.

Culture: 24hour cultures of *Pseudomonas aeruginosa and Escherichia coli.*

Instrument Required

Test tube, Inoculating loop, Autoclave, Filtration assembly, Whatman filter paper, laminar airflow cabinet and Incubator.

Procedure

1. The bacterial culture is inoculated with help of inoculating needle in the Hugh and Leifson's Oxidative Fermentation Basal Agar tube aseptically by means of stabbing four or five times to a depth of 2.5cm.

2. Inoculate the bacteria in a control tube without carbohydrate for comparison.

3. Incubate for 7 days at 30°C.

4. Observe the results

   (a) If the media turns to yellow color – Acid formation happened pH 6.0 (Positive reaction) – fermenter generally turns entire tube yellow in 18hrs, where us oxidizers turns top half of the tube yellow.

   (b) If the media turns yellow – green to green when compared to control which is more alkaline formation happened. (weak reaction)

   (c) If the media remains no change in color with control – Negative reaction

Observation

S. No.	Characterization	Observation
1	Color of the top of the medium	

Report

Chapter 20

Kligler's Iron Agar Test

Object

1. To understand the biochemical basis of Kligler's Iron Agar Test.
2. To perform Kligler's Iron Agar Test.

Principle

This test is performed for the determination of the ability of fastidious organism to ferment glucose, which gives negative results to oxidative fermentation medium (see carbohydrate utilization test). The production H_2S will help for the identification of *Erysipelothrix* and *Campylobacter*.

Kligler's Iron Agar (KIA) contains casein and meat peptone and 0.1% glucose & 1% lactose for fermentation and the change in pH is identified by phenol red indicator present in the medium. The ferrous and ferric ions & sodium thio sulphate is added in the medium to identify the production of hydrogen sulfide.

Organism that is not lactose fermenting initially produce the yellow color because of the production of acid from glucose, latter on the oxidative metabolism continues in the media leads to the breakdown of peptone and change the color form yellow to red (converts acid to alkali). If there is no oxygen penetration in the media than the butt remains yellow because of no oxidative metabolism.

By this test we can categorize the bacteria in the following types.

1. The non lactose fermenting organism yields a red slant with yellow butt (alkaline slant over acid butt).
2. So lactose fermenting organism will remain yellow both slant and butt (continue acid production)
3. Non fermenting organism will give red color to both slant and butt (no acid production)

The gas production in the media is identified by the presence of bubbles or rupturing of the medium. If the gas produced is H_2S is identified by the reduction of ferric ion, which produces a black precipitate.

Material Required

Culture: 24 hour cultures of *Escherichia coli* (A/A + gas), *Proteus mirabilis* (K/A + H_2S), *Pseudomonas aeruginosa* (K/K, no gas), *Salmonella typhimurium* (K/A + H_2S+ gas),

Medium: Kligler's Iron Agar Medium

Table 20.1

S. No.	Composition	Amount for 1000 mL
1	Enzymatic Digest of Casein	10.0 gm
2	Enzymatic Digest of Animal Tissue	10.0 gm
3	Lactose	10.0 gm
4	Dextrose	1.0 gm
5	Ferric Ammonium Citrate	0.5 gm
6	Sodium Chloride	5.0 gm
7	Sodium Thiosulfate	0.5 gm
8	Phenol Red	0.025 gm
9	Agar	15.0 gm
10	Distill Water	1000 mL
pH – 7.4 ± 0.2 at 25ºC		

Autoclave at 121ºC for 15 minutes

Instrument required

Inoculating loop and needle, Autoclave, laminar airflow cabinet and Incubator.

Procedure

1. The bacterial culture is inoculated with help of inoculating needle in Kligler's Iron Agar tube aseptically by means of stabbing within 3 to 5 mm from the bottom of the tube.

2. Withdraw the needle and streak the entire surface of the slant.

3. Incubate for 18 to 24hrs at 35 to 37°C.

4. Observe the results for the color of the slant and butt.

5. Observe for gas and hydrogen sulphide production.

Observation

S. No.	Characterization	Observation
1	Color of the slant	
2	Color of the Butt	
3	Gas production	
4	H_2S production	

Report

Chapter 21

Triple Sugar Iron Agar Test

Object

1. To understand the biochemical basis of Triple Sugar Iron Agar Test.
2. To perform Triple Sugar Iron Agar Test.

Principle

This test is performed for the determination of the ability of fastidious organism to ferment glucose, which gives negative results to oxidative fermentation medium (see carbohydrate utilization test). The production H_2S will help for the identification of *Erysipelothrix* and *Campylobacter*.

Triple Sugar Iron Agar (TSI) contains casein and meat peptone and triple carbohydrate source 0.1% glucose, 1% sucrose & 1% lactose for fermentation and the change in pH is identified by phenol red indicator present in the medium. The ferrous and ferric ions & sodium thio sulphate is added in the medium to identify the production of hydrogen sulfide.

Based on carbohydrate utilization and hydrogen sulfide production, a TSI slant can be interpreted in several ways:

1. **Glucose Fermenting Microorganism:** If the tube reaction is alkaline slant over acid butt (K/A) signifying that only glucose is metabolized. The bacteria quickly metabolized the glucose, initially producing an acid slant and an acid butt (A/A) in a few hours. After further incubation (more than 18 hours) the glucose was consumed, and because the bacteria could not use lactose or sucrose, the peptones were utilized as an energy source aerobically, on the slant causes the release of ammonia (NH3), which turn pH alkaline turning from yellow to red color to the slant. In the butt, the bacteria use the glucose and forms stable acid end product, thus the butt remains acidic.

The example of the bacteria producing a K/A reaction with or without gas include: *Citrobacter freundii* , *Citrobacter koseri*, and *Morganella morganii.*

2. **Glucose, Lactose and/or Sucrose Fermenter:** If the tube reaction is acid slant over acid butt (A/A) indicating that glucose, lactose and/or sucrose have been metabolized. The bacteria quickly metabolized the glucose, producing an acid slant and an acid butt in a few hours. On further incubation (after 18 hours) the glucose was consumed, and then the bacteria continue to utilized lactose and/or sucrose as energy source, maintaining an acid slant. The results are recorded as acid over acid (A/A). If the medium still incubated longer, more than 48 hours, the lactose and sucrose would be depleted, and the slant would revert to an alkaline pH due to metabolism of the peptones.

   The example of the bacteria commonly producing an A/A reaction with or without gas include: *Enterobacter aerogenes, E. cloacae, Escherichia coli, Klebsiella oxytoca,* and *K. pneumoniae.*

3. **Glucose, Lactose and Sucrose Nonfermenters:** If the tube reaction is either alkaline slant over alkaline butt (K/K) or alkaline slant over no change (K/NC) indicating that all three sugars have not been metabolized. The difference between K/K and K/NC is subtle. Some non-enteric bacteria, such as the *pseudomonas,* are unable to ferment glucose, lactose, or sucrose. These bacteria derive energy from peptones either aerobically or anaerobically. Non-glucose fermenter's can produce two possible reactions. If the bacteria can metabolize peptones both aerobically and anaerobically, the slant and butt will be red (alkaline over alkaline; K/K). If peptones can only be metabolized aerobically, the slant will be red and the butt will exhibit no change (K/NC). Bacteria producing K/K or K/NC

   The example of the bacteria commonly producing an K/K and K/NC reaction with or without gas *Acinetobacter* spp. and *Pseudomonas* spp.

The gas production in the media is identified by the presence of bubbles or rupturing of the medium. If the gas produced is H_2S is identified by the reduction of ferric ion, which produces a black precipitate.

Material Required

Culture: 24hour cultures of *Escherichia coli* (A/A + gas), *Proteus mirabilis* (K/A + H_2S), *Pseudomonas aeruginosa* (K/K, no gas), *Salmonella typhimurium* (K/A + H_2S+ gas) and *Shigella flexneri* (K/A + no H_2S + no gas).

Medium: Triple Sugar Iron Agar Medium.

Table 21.1

S. No.	Composition	Amount for 1000 mL
1	Enzymatic Digest of Casein	5.0 gm
2	Enzymatic Digest of Animal Tissue	5.0 gm
3	Yeast enriched peptone	10.0 gm
4	Sucrose	10.0 gm
5	Lactose	10.0 gm
6	Dextrose	1.0 gm
7	Ferric Ammonium Citrate	0.2 gm
8	Sodium Chloride	5.0 gm
9	Sodium Thiosulfate	0.3 gm
10	Phenol Red	0.025 gm
11	Agar	13.5gm
12	Distill Water	1000 mL
pH – 7.3 ± 0.2 at 25°C		

Autoclave at 121 °C for 15 minutes

Instrument required

Inoculating loop and needle, autoclave, laminar airflow cabinet and incubator

Procedure

1. The bacterial culture is inoculated with help of inoculating needle in Triple sugar Iron Agar tube aseptically by means of stabbing within 3 to 5 mm from the bottom of the tube.

2. Withdraw the needle and streak the entire surface of the slant.

3. Incubate for 18 to 24 hrs at 35 to 37 °C.

4. Observe the results for the color of the slant and butt

5. Observe for gas and hydrogen sulphide production.

Observation

S. No.	Characterization	Observation
1	Color of the slant	
2	Color of the Butt	
3	Gas production	
4	H_2S production	

Report

Chapter 22

Indole Production Test (IMViC Test)

Object

1. To understand the biochemical basis of Indole Production Test.
2. To perform Indole Production Test.

Principle

This test is performed for the determination of the ability of a micro organism to degrade the amino acid tryptophan and produce indole. It is used as part of the IMViC procedures, a series of tests designed to distinguish among members of the family Enterobacteriaceae.

The bacteria containing the enzyme tryptophanase causes the amino acid Tryptophan to undergo deamination and hydrolysis with the formation of indole, pyruvic acid and ammonia.

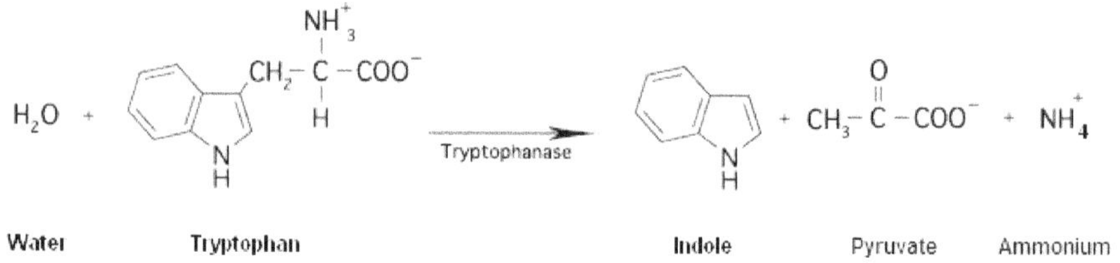

The production of indole is identified by its reaction with Kovac's Reagent (which contains hydrochloric acid and dimethy laminobenzaldehyde in amyl alcohol), the solution turns from yellow to cherry red.

Material Required

Culture: 24 hour cultures of Escherichia coli and Enterobacter aerogenes.

Medium: Sulfide-indole-motility (SIM Agar) medium

S. No.	Composition	Amount for 1000 mL
1	Peptone	30.0 gm
2	Beef extract	3.0 gm
3	Ferrous ammonium sulfate	0.2 gm
4	Sodium thiosulfate	0.025 gm
5	Agar	3.0 gm
6	Distill Water	1000 mL

pH – 7.3 ± 0.2 at 25ºC

Autoclave at 121ºC for 15 minutes, prepare deep tubes.

Instrument Required

Inoculating loop and needle, Autoclave, laminar airflow cabinet and Incubator.

Procedure

1. The bacterial culture is inoculated with help of inoculating needle in SIM Agar deep tube aseptically by means of stabbing approximately two-thirds of the way into the deep.
2. Incubate for 24 to 42 hrs at 35 to 37°C.
3. 5 drops of Kovac's reagent should be added to the top of the tube
4. A positive test is indicated by the formation of a red color in the reagent layer on top of the agar deep tube within seconds of adding the reagent.
5. If the test is negative, the reagent layer will remain yellow or be slightly cloudy.

Observation

S. No.	Characterization	Observation
1	Color	
2	Indole production	

Report

Chapter 23

MR-VP (Methyl Red-Voges Proskauer) Test (IMViC Test)

Object

1. To understand the biochemical basis of methyl red – Voges Proskauer test.
2. To perform methyl red – Voges Proskauer test.

Principle

This test is a part of the IMViC procedures, a series of tests designed to distinguish among members of the family *Enterobacteriaceae*.

Methyl Red Test: This test is performed to determine the microorganism has a ability to form a stable acid end product from glucose fermentation. All microorganisms belonging to the family Enterobacteriaceae gives a positive methyl red test upto 24hrs. Those organisms which will continue to metabolize the pyruvic acid further to lactic, acetic and formic acids by mixed acid pathways are able to maintain the pH <4.4. Organisms which follow other pathways like butylene Glycol pathway produces acetoin and butanediol, which are neutral end products shows pH 6.0. The reduction in pH is identified by the methyl red indicator which give red color at pH< 4.4 and yellow at pH >6.0.

Voges Proskauer Test: This test is performed to identify the microorganism has an ability to produce acetylmethylcarbinol (acetoin) from glucose. The formation of acetylmethylcarbinol is identified by the addition of strong alkali like 40% Potassium Hydroxide, which converts acetoin into diacetyl by the action of 40% KOH and atmospheric oxygen. The formed diacetyl and the Quinidine containing compounds present in the peptone (media) form pinkish red polymer. The indensity of the color can be raised by the addition of α- napthol.

Material Required

Culture: 24 hour cultures of *Escherichia coli* (MR – Negative, VP-positive) and *Klebsiella pneumonia* (MR – positive, VP - Negative).

Medium: MRVP Broth medium.

S. No.	Composition	Amount for 1000 mL
1	Buffered Peptone	7.0 gm
2	Glucose	5.0 gm
3	Di potassium phosphate	5.0 gm
4	Distill Water	1000 mL
pH – 6.9 ± 0.2 at 25°C		

Autoclave at 121 °C for 15 minutes, prepare deep tubes.

Instrument Required

Inoculating loop and needle, Autoclave, laminar airflow cabinet and Incubator.

Methyl Red Test Procedure

1. The bacterial culture is inoculated in MRVP broth tube aseptically.
2. It is incubated for 48hrs at 35 to 37°C.
3. Add 3 to 6 drops of methyl red indicator.
4. Observe the formation of red color immediately.

Voges Proskauer Test Procedure

1. The bacterial culture is inoculated in MRVP broth tube aseptically.
2. It is incubated for 18 to 24hrs at 35 to 37°C.
3. Add 6 drops of α-napthol and mix well.
4. Then add 2 drops of 40% KOH and mix well.
5. Shake well for 30 minutes and observe the formation of pink red color at surface for positive reaction.

Observation

S. No.	Characterization	Observation
1	Color – MR Test	
2	Color – VP Test	

Report

Chapter 24

Citrate Utilization Test (Simmon Citrate Test) (IMViC Test)

Object

1. To understand the biochemical basis of Citrate Utilization test.
2. To perform Citrate Utilization test.

Principle

This test is a part of the IMViC procedures, a series of tests designed to distinguish among members of the family *Enterobacteriaceae*.

This test is performed to determine the ability of the microorganism to utilize citrate as an energy source. The microorganism Salmonella, Citrobacter, Klebsiella, Enterobacter, Edwardsiella, Providencia and Serratia gives positive results and Shigella, Escherichia, Yersinia and Morganella gives negative results.

The medium contains citrate as sole carbon source and inorganic ammonium salts as source of nitrogen. The bacteria which can utilize the citrate through Krebs cycle (an intermediate metabolite) liberate ammonia by means of breakdown of ammonium salts, which alters the pH to go above 7.6. The change is pH is identified by the Bromthymol blue indicator turns green to blue color of the medium.

Material Required

Culture: 24 hour cultures of *Escherichia coli* (Negative) and *Klebsiella pneumonia* (Positive).

Medium: Simmon Citrate Agar medium.

Table 24.1

S. No.	Composition	Amount for 1000 mL
1	Ammonium Dihydrogen Phosphate	1.0 gm
2	Di potassium Phosphate	1.0 gm
3	Sodium Chloride	5.0 gm
4	Sodium Citrate	2.0 gm
5	Magnesium Sulfate	0.2 gm
6	Bromthymol Blue	0.08 gm
7	Agar	15.0 gm
8	Distill Water	1000 ml
pH – 6.9 ± 0.2 at 25°C		

Autoclave at 121°C for 15 minutes, prepare deep tubes

Instrument Required

Inoculating loop and needle, autoclave, laminar airflow cabinet and Incubator.

Procedure

1. The bacterial culture is inoculated in Simmon Citrate Agar slant tube aseptically by streaking back and forth.
2. Incubate for 4 days at 35 to 37 °C.
3. Observe the color change green to blue along the slant.

Observation

S. No.	Characterization	Observation
1	Color of the slant	

Report

Chapter 25

Hydrogen Sulfide Production Test

Object

1. To understand the biochemical basis of Hydrogen Sulfide Production Test.
2. To perform Hydrogen Sulfide Production Test.

Principle

All members of the family *Enterobacteriaceae* are capable of producing various amounts of H_2S.

The microorganism *Erysipelothrix* and fastidious gram negative rods like *Campylobacter* gives positive results.

This test is performed to check the ability of the microorganism to liberate H_2S either by enzymatically liberating sulfur from inorganic sulfur as H_2S or proteolytic degradation of sulfur containing amino acids.

The bacteria reacts with the sodium thiosulfate present in the medium to yield sulfite and H_2S, the produced H_2S reacts with the ferric ion or lead acetate to yield ferrous sulfide or lead sulfide forms an insoluble black precipitate.

Material Required

Culture: 24 hour cultures of *Escherichia coli* (Negative) and *Campylobacter* (positive).

Medium: Sulfide-indole-motility (SIM Agar) medium.

S. No.	Composition	Amount for 1000 mL
1	Peptone	30.0 gm
2	Beef extract	3.0 gm
3	Ferrous ammonium sulfate	0.2 gm
4	Sodium thiosulfate	0.025 gm

Table *Contd...*

S. No.	Composition	Amount for 1000 mL
5	Agar	3.0 gm
6	Distill Water	1000 mL
pH – 7.3 ± 0.2 at 25ºC		

Autoclave at 121ºC for 15 minutes, prepare deep tubes

Instrument Required

Inoculating loop and needle, Autoclave, laminar airflow cabinet and Incubator.

Procedure

1. The bacterial culture is inoculated in SIM Agar deep tube aseptically by stabbing the inoculating needle to within 3 to 5mm from the bottom of the tube.
2. Incubate for 18 to 24hrs (sometimes up to 3days) at 35 to 37°C.
3. Observe the black precipitate indicating hydrogen sulfide production.

Observation

S. No.	Characterization	Observation
1	Presence of Black precipitate	

Report

Chapter 26

Glucan and Polysaccharide Production Test

Object

1. To understand the biochemical basis of Glucan and Polysaccharide Production test.
2. To perform Glucan and Polysaccharide Production test.

Principle

The Glucan production test is performed to identify the *Streptococci*, which has an ability to produce glucans (an extracellular polysaccharide) from sucrose. The type of *streptococci* species can be identified by the type of glucans produced (Slim adherence etc).

The Polysaccharide production test is used to identify some saprophytic *Nesseria species* can produce and iodine reacting polysaccharide from sucrose with the help of amylosucrase enzyme.

Both glucans and polysaccharide form brown to black color when iodine is added to the medium.

Material Required

Culture for Glucans: 24hour cultures of *Streptococci bovis* (Positive) and *Enterococcus faecalis* (Negative).

Culture for Polysaccharides: 24hour cultures of *Neisseria polysaccharea* (Positive) and *Neisseria gonorrhoeae* (Negative).

Medium: Heart Infusion Agar medium.

S. No.	Composition	Amount for 1000 mL
1	Infusion from Beef Heart	500.0 gm
2	Tryptose	10.0 gm
3	Sodium Chloride	5.0 gm

Table Contd...

S. No.	Composition	Amount for 1000 mL
4	Agar	15.0 gm
6	Distill Water	1000 mL
pH – 7.4 ± 0.2 at 25 ᵒC		

Autoclave at 121ᵒC for 15 minutes, prepare petri plates

Instrument Required

Inoculating loop and needle, Autoclave, laminar airflow cabinet and Incubator.

Procedure

1. The bacterial culture is inoculated in Heart Infusion Agar medium aseptically by streaking the petri plates.
2. Incubate for 24 to 48hrs (without CO_2) at 35 to 37°C.
3. Observe colonies for Glucan production.
4. Add 2 drops of iodine solution and observe the dark reddish brown to black precipitate for polysaccharide production.

Observation

S. No.	Characterization	Observation
1	Presence of Glucan	
2	Color of the precipitate	

Report

Chapter 27

Gelatin Liquefaction Test (Kohn Method)

Object

1. To understand the biochemical basis of Gelatin Liquefaction Test.
2. To perform Gelatin Liquefaction Test.

Principle

Gelatin test is useful for the identification of gram negative rods for the separation of fluorescent *Pseudomonas* and gram positive rods for the identification of species.

The organism which has the capable of producing the enzyme Gelatinases can hydrolyze the gelatin into polypeptides and individual amino acids, so the gelatin loses its characteristic state and gets liquefied.

Material Required

Culture: 24 hour cultures of *Pseudomonas aeruginosa* (Positive) and *Escherichia coli* (Negative).

Medium: Kohn Gelatin Charcoal medium

Table 27.1

S. No.	Composition	Amount for 1000 mL
1	Peptone	5.0 gm
2	Beef Extract	3.0 gm
3	Nutrient Gelatin	150.0 gm
4	Powdered Charcoal	30.0 to 50.0 gm
5	Distill Water	1000 ml
pH – 6.8 ± 0.2 at 25ºC		

Autoclave at 121ºC for 15 minutes, prepare petri plates.

Instrument Required

Inoculating loop and needle, Autoclave, laminar airflow cabinet and Incubator.

Procedure

1. The bacterial culture is inoculated in Kohn Gelatin Charcoal medium deep tube aseptically by stabbing the inoculating needle to within 3 to 5mm from the bottom of the tube. Similarly prepare an un-inoculated culture tube also.

2. Incubate for 1 week at 25 to 27 °C.

3. Observe the liquefaction and further its liquefaction in confirmed by keeping the tubes in ice bath for 15 to 30 minutes.

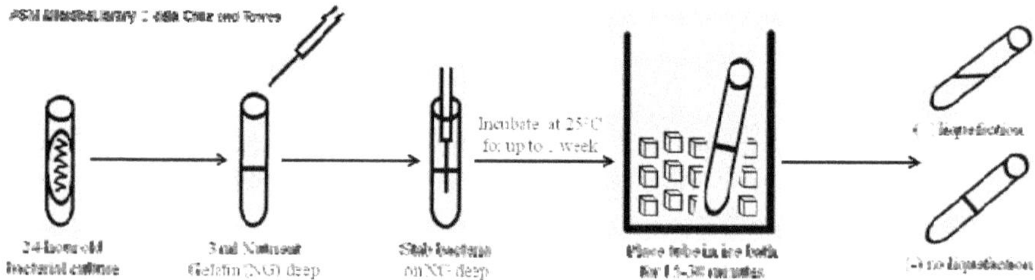

Fig. 27.1 Gelatin Liquefaction Test (Kohn Method).

Observation

S. No.	Characterization	Observation
1	Liquefaction of gelatin tube	

Report

Chapter 28

Tube Coagulase Test

Object

1. To understand the biochemical basis of Coagulase Test.
2. To perform Coagulase Test.

Principle

This test is performed for the identification of pathogenic staphylococci like *staphylococcus aureus* in humans, *staphylococcus intermedius* in dogs, *staphylococcus delphini* in dolphins, *staphylococcus lutrae* from otters *and staphylococcus hyicus* from pigs.

These microorganisms secrete the enzyme Coagulase is a thermo-stable thrombin like substance that activates the fibrinogen to form fibrin resulting in a clot. This is identified by inoculating the microorganism in a test tube containing plasma. The free Coagulase is liberated and forms the clot, sometimes the bounded Coagulase or clumping factor bound to cell surface receptor has the ability to act directly on the fibrinogen in plasma to form clump.

Material Required

Culture: 24hour cultures of *staphylococcus aureus* (Positive) and *Escherichia coli* (Negative).

Chemical required: Rabbit plasma.

Instrument required: Inoculating loop and needle, Autoclave, laminar airflow cabinet and Incubator.

Procedure

1. Two test tubes are taken and labeled with respective microorganism name.
2. Each tube is filled with 1 mL of 1 in 10 diluted rabbit plasma.
3. To the tube respective microorganism where inoculated.
4. All the tubes are incubated at 37 ºC.

5. Observe the suspensions at half hourly intervals for a period of four hours.

6. Positive result is indicated by gelling of the plasma, which remains in place even after inverting the tube.

7. If the test remains negative until four hours at 37 ºC, the tube is kept at room temperature for overnight incubation.

Observation

S. No.	Characterization	Observation
1	Formation of Clot	

Report

Chapter 29

Decarboxylase-Dihydrolase Test

Object

1. To understand the biochemical basis of Decarboxylase-Dihydrolase Test.
2. To perform Decarboxylase-Dihydrolase Test.

Principle

This test is performed to detect the ability of the microorganism to decarboxylate or hydrolyze an amino acid. It is performed for the identification of enteric gram negative rods and *Vibrio, Plesiomonas* and *Aeromonas* at species level.

The Arginine, lysine and ornithine is decarboxylated or hydrolyzed to form an amine that produces an alkaline pH, which is identified by the pH indicators bromcresol purple and cresol red.

The media contains meat peptones and beef extract as nitrogen source, glucose as carbohydrate source and Arginine, lysine & ornithine are amino acid source is added in the medium to detect the production of the enzyme which decarboxylate or hydrolyze these substrates. Pyridoxal is added as enzyme cofactor which enhance the decarboxylase activity. Initially because of the fermentation of the carbohydrate the media changes the color from purple to yellow (lowering of pH), if the decarboxylation or hydrolysis of amino acid causes the color change to purple (increase in pH because of formation of amine – alkaline region).

On decarboxylation of arginine forms agmatine, lysine forms cadaverine and ornithine forms putrescine. The agmatine can be further hydrolyzed to putrescine. The arginine is also hydrolyzed directly by arginine dehyrolase to form citrulline.

Material Required

Culture: 24hour cultures of following cultures.

Table 29.1

S. No.	Microorganism name	Arginine	Lysine	Ornithine
1	*Klebsiella pneumonia*	Negative	Positive	Negative
2	*Enterobacter cloacae*	Positive	Negative	Positive
3	*Staphylococcus aureus*	NA	NA	Negative
4	*Staphylococcus lugdunensis*	NA	NA	Positive

Medium: Moeller Decarboxylase Broth Base medium

Table 29.2

S. No.	Composition	Amount for 1000 mL
1	Peptic Digest of Animal Tissue	5.0 gm
2	Beef Extract	5.0 gm
3	Bromcresol Purple	0.01 gm
4	Cresol Red	0.005 gm
5	Dextrose	0.5 gm
6	Pyridoxal .	0.005 gm
7	Distill Water	1000 mL
pH – 6.0 ± 0.2 at 25ºC		

Add 1% of Arginine, lysine & ornithine for the respective test protocols

Autoclave at 121ºC for 15 minutes, prepare petri plates.

Chemical required: Mineral oil and liquid paraffin or petroleum jelly maintained in liquid form.

Instrument required: Inoculating loop and needle, Autoclave, laminar airflow cabinet and Incubator.

Procedure

1. Take the necessary quantity of test tubes and mark with the media with type of amino acid and microorganism to be inoculated.

2. Inoculate each marked broth media by transferring one or two colonies from the surface of a fresh culture with an inoculating loop or needle of respective microorganism.

3. Mix well to distribute the culture throughout the medium.

4. Overlay the medium in each tube with 1 mL sterile mineral oil and liquid paraffin or petroleum jelly (to maintain anaerobic condition – favors decarboxylation activity).

5. Incubate the tubes with caps tightened at 35 ± 2°C.

6. Examine for growth and decarboxylase reactions after 18–24, 48, 72 and 96 h before reporting as negative.

7. The medium will become yellow initially, if the dextrose is fermented, and then will gradually turn purple.

8. If the decarboxylase reaction occurs and elevates the pH.

Observation

S. No.	Characterization	Observation			
		Base media	**1% Arginine**	**1% Lysine**	**1% Ornithine**
1	Initial Color of the media				
2	Final color of the media				
3	Test Result				

Report

Chapter 30

Centrimide Test

Object

1. To understand the biochemical basis of Cetrimide Test.
2. To perform Cetrimide Test.

Principle

This test is performed to identify the microorganism to *Pseudomonas aeruginosa*.

The Cetrimide is a quaternary ammonium salt (detergent) used as a disinfectant, most of the bacteria are killed by its germicidal action by means of release of nitrogen and phosphorus are released form bacterial cell when it comes in contact. The growth of the bacteria is the positive result for this test in a slant media containing magnesium chloride and potassium sulfate. The *Pseudomonas aeruginosa* enhances the production of pyocyanin and pyoverdin (fluorescein) from magnesium chloride and potassium sulfate.

Material Required

Culture: 24 hour cultures of *Pseudomonas aeruginosa* (Positive) and *E coli* (Negative).

Medium: Cetrimide Agar Medium.

S. No.	Composition	Amount for 1000 mL
1	Pancreatic Digest of Gelatin	20.0 gm
2	Magnesium Chloride	1.4 gm
3	Potassium Sulfate	10.0 gm
4	Cetrimide (Cetyl tri methyl ammonium Bromide).	0.3 gm
5	Agar	13.6 gm
7	Distill Water	1000 mL
pH – 7.2 ± 0.2 at 25ºC		

Autoclave at 121 ºC for 15 minutes, Supplement – 10 mL of Glycerol for 1 L of media

Instrument Required

Inoculating loop and needle, Autoclave, UV light chamber, laminar airflow cabinet and Incubator.

Procedure

1. Take the necessary quantity of test tubes and mark with the media with microorganism to be inoculated.
2. Inoculate the microorganism in the slant by means of streaking back and forth ascetically.
3. Incubate aerobically at 35 ± 2°C for up to 7 days.
4. Observe the growth and pigment.
5. If no pigment is visible, observe under UV light.
6. If negative for pigment at 24hr, incubate in dark at 25ºC to enhance the pigmentation.

Observation

S. No.	Characterization	Observation
1	Growth of the organism	
2	Pigmentation on naked eye	
3	Pigmentation under UV light	

Report

Chapter 31

Catalase Test

Object

1. To understand the biochemical basis of Catalase Test.
2. To perform Catalase Test.

Principle

This test is performed to check the ability of the microorganism to produce the enzyme Catalase. It is primarily useful in differentiating between genera of catalase-positive *Micrococcaceae* from catalase-negative *Streptococcaceae* and species of certain gram positives such as *Aerococcus urinae* (positive) from *Aerococcus viridians* (negative).

The catalase enzyme serves to neutralize the bactericidal effects of hydrogen peroxide by hydrolyzing it to water and oxygen ($2H_2O_2 +$ Catalase $\rightarrow 2H_2O + O_2$). This results in the rapid liberation of gas bubbles.

Material Required

Culture: 24 hour cultures of *Staphylococcus aureus* (Positive) and *E coli* (Negative).

Chemical required: 3% hydrogen peroxide, for others use more than 15% H_2O_2.

Instrument Required

Inoculating loop, needle and glass slide.

Procedure

1. Take a clean glass slide and place the microorganism at the center of slide, which is visible in the naked eye.
2. Place a drop of Hydrogen Peroxide and immediately observe the effervescence, use magnifying glass in necessary.

Observation

S. No.	Characterization	Observation
1	Presence of air bubble	

Report

Chapter 32

Leucine Aminopeptidase Test (LAP Test)

Object

1. To understand the biochemical basis of Leucine Aminopepdidase Test (LAP Test).
2. To perform Leucine Aminopepdidase Test (LAP Test).

Principle

This test is performed to check the ability of the microorganism to produce the enzyme Leucine Aminopepdidase. It is used for identification of the catalase negative gram positive cocci and to differentiate LAP positive *Streptococcus, Enterococcus, lactococcus and Pediococcus* from *Aerococcus* and *Leuconostoc.*

The bacteria secreting the enzyme Leucine Aminopepdidase hydrolyze the substrate Leucine-p-naphthylamide to release free Leucine and β-naphthylamide. The β-naphthylamide combines with cinnamaldehyde reagent to produce cherry red pigment from pink.

Material Required

Culture: 18hour cultures of *Enterococcus faecalis* (Positive) and *Aerococcus viridians* (Negative).

Chemical required: LAP Test Disks.

Instrument Required

Inoculating loop and needle, Autoclave, laminar airflow cabinet and Incubator.

Procedure

1. Place the disk in a Petri dish, moisten with a loop full of distilled water.

2. Inoculate the microorganism in the disk ascetically.
3. Incubate at room temperature for 5 minutes.
4. Add 1 drop of cinnamaldehyde and wait for 2 minute to observe the color change.

Observation

S. No.	Characterization	Observation
1	Color change after 2 min	

Report

Chapter 33

Malonate Test

Object

1. To understand the biochemical basis of Malonate Test.
2. To perform Malonate Test.

Principle

This test is performed for differentiating the microorganism to *Enterobacteriaceae* and especially *Klebsiella and Salmonella*.

Malonate is a succinic acid inhibitor, which inhibits the Krebs and glycolytic cycle. The bacteria will only survive and grow if it has the ability to utilize malonate as carbon source. The positive result is identified by the bacterial fermentation of sodium malonate to form sodium hydroxide and sodium bi carbonate, which increase the pH in alkaline region and it is indicated by the bromthymol blue indicator turns the color of the media from green to blue. Malonate negative bacteria utilize the glucose from the media and forms acid end product, which turns the media to yellow color.

Material Required

Culture: 24 hour cultures of *Klebsiella pneumoniae* (Positive) and *E coli* (Negative).

Medium: Malonate Broth Medium.

S. No	Composition	Amount for 1000 mL
1	Yeast Extract	1.0 gm
2	Ammonium Sulfate	2.0 gm
3	Dipotassium Phosphate	0.6 gm
4	Monopotassium Phosphate	0.4 gm
5	Sodium Chloride	2.0 gm
6	Sodium malonate	3.0 gm
7	Glucose	0.25 gm
8	Bromthymol blue	0.025 gm
9	Deionized Water	1000 mL
pH – 6.7 ± 0.2 at 25°C		

Autoclave at 121°C for 15 minutes.

Instrument Required

Inoculating loop and needle, autoclave, laminar airflow cabinet and incubator.

Procedure

1. Take the necessary quantity of test tubes and mark with the media with microorganism to be inoculated.
2. Inoculate the microorganism in the broth ascetically.
3. Incubate aerobically at 35 ± 2°C for up to 48hrs.
4. Observe the growth and color change from green to blue.

Observation

S. No.	Characterization	Observation
1	Growth of the organism	
2	Color of the media	

Report

Chapter 34

Methyl Glucopyranoside Test (MGP Test)

Object

1. To understand the biochemical basis of Methyl Glucopyranoside Test (MGP Test).
2. To perform Methyl Glucopyranoside Test (MGP Test).

Principle

This test is performed for differentiating *Enterococci* based on the ability to acidify the carbohydrate methyl-α-D-glucopyranoside, which is identified by the yellow color change of the media by the pH indicator phenol red.

This test is useful for preventing the misidentification of vancomycin resistant *Enterococcus gallinarum* as vancomycin resistant *Enterococcus faecium*.

Material Required

Culture: 24 hour cultures of *Enterococcus gallinarum* (Positive – yellow color of the media) and *Enterococcus faecium*. (Negative – red or orange color of the media).

Medium: Methyl Glucopyranoside Broth Medium (MGP Broth).

Table 34.1

S. No	Composition	Amount for 1000 mL
1	Pancreatic digest of casein	10.0 gm
2	Sodium Chloride	5.0 gm
3	Methyl Glucopyranoside	10.0 gm
4	Phenol red	18.0 mg
5	Deionized Water	1000 mL
pH – 7.4 ± 0.2 at 25ºC		

Autoclave at 121ºC for 15 minutes.

Instrument Required

Inoculating loop and needle, autoclave, laminar airflow cabinet and incubator.

Procedure

1. Take the necessary quantity of test tubes and mark with the media with microorganism to be inoculated.
2. Inoculate the microorganism in the broth ascetically.
3. Incubate aerobically at 35 ± 2°C for 24 hrs.
4. Observe the yellow color change of the media.

Observation

S. No.	Characterization	Observation
1	Color of the media	

Report

Chapter 35

Nitrate/Nitrate Reduction Test

Object

1. To understand the biochemical basis of Nitrate/Nitrate Reduction Test.
2. To perform Nitrate/Nitrate Reduction Test.

Principle

This test is performed for differentiating *Moraxella catarrhalis from Neisseria* based on the ability to reduce nitrate and nitrites. This test is also useful for the evaluation of non-glucose fermenting and fastidious gram negative rods.

The Nitrate and nitrite broth are used for the detection of the ability of microorganism to reduce nitrate to nitrite and nitrite to reduce further.

The end products of the nitrate reduction are nitrite, ammonia, molecular nitrogen, hydroxyl amine etc. The Nitrite is detected by the formation of red diazonium compound when it reacts with sulfanilic acid and α-naphthylamine. The nitrogen gas is detected by its entrapment in the durham tube present in the broth. This test is positive for Nitrate reduction only.

Both Nitrate and Nitrite reduction is detected by adding zinc dust if nitrate and nitrites both reduced to nitrogen compounds no red color develops. If the nitrate is not utilized it will be reduced by the zinc to nitrite which is detected as red color – negative.

Material Required

Culture: 24 hour cultures of *Pseudomonas aeruginosa* (Positive – nitrate and gas) and *Acinetobacter baumannii.* (Negative – nitrate)

Medium: Nitrate Broth Medium.

S. No	Composition	Amount for 1000 mL
1	Peptone	20.0 gm
2	Potassium nitrate	2.0 gm
3	Deionized Water	1000 mL
pH – 7.4 ± 0.2 at 25ºC		

Autoclave at 121ºC for 15 minutes.

Medium: Nitrite Broth Medium.

S. No	Composition	Amount for 1000 mL
1	Heart infusion broth	25.0 gm
2	Potassium nitrate	0.1 to 1.0 gm
3	Deionized Water	1000 mL
pH – 7.4 ± 0.2 at 25ºC		

Autoclave at 121ºC for 15 minutes.

Chemical Required

Reagent A (0.8% Sulfanilic acid) – add 0.8 gm of Sulfanilic acid in 70 mL of distill water and heat to dissolve, add 30 ml of glacial acetic acid after cooling.

Reagent B (0.5% N,N- Dimethyl-α-naphthylamine) – mix 30 mL of glacial acetic acid and 70 mL of distilled water to this add 0.5gm of N, N- Dimethyl-α-naphthylamine.

Instrument Required

Inoculating loop and needle, autoclave, laminar airflow cabinet and incubator.

Procedure

1. Take the necessary quantity of test tubes and mark with the media with microorganism to be inoculated.
2. Place the Durham tube inside the broth tube ascetically without the entrapment of gas bubble.
3. Inoculate the microorganism in the broth ascetically.
4. Incubate aerobically at 35 ± 2°C for 2 to 5 days.
5. Observe the gas in the Durham's vial and growth of the bacteria. (if there is no growth don't add the reagents)

6. If growth of microorganism is there add 2 to 3 drops of reagent A and mix well by tapping or shaking the tube, then add 2 to 3 drops of reagent B and mix well.

7. Observe the red color development within 1 to 2 minutes.

Observation

S. No.	Characterization	Observation
1	Growth of the microorganism	
2	Color of the media	
3	Presence of gas in Durham tube	

Report

Chapter 36

Oxidase Test

Object

1. To understand the biochemical basis of Oxidase Test.
2. To perform Oxidase Test.

Principle

This test is used for the initial characterization of gram negative bacteria especially *Pseudomonadaceae* from *Enterobacteriaceae*. The bacteria intracellular cytochrome oxidase enzyme oxidizes the tetramethyl-p-phenylenediamine dihydrochloride to purple color compound indophenol blue.

Material Required

Culture: 24 hour cultures of *Pseudomonas aeruginosa* (Positive) and *E.coli.* (Negative).

Chemical Required

Kovac's Reagent (0.5% to 1.0%) – dissolve 1.0 gm of N, N, N, N tetramethyl-p-phenylenediamine dihydrochloride in 10 mL of sterile distill wate, mix well and wait for 10 minutes.

Instrument Required

Sterile paper disk, Inoculating loop and needle, autoclave, laminar airflow cabinet and incubator.

Procedure: Filter Paper Method

1. Place a square of Whatman filter paper No 1 in a petri dish.
2. Moisten the filter paper with 1 to 2 drops of Kovacs reagent.
3. Inoculate the bacteria in filter paper.

4. Observe the development of purple color within 10 to 30 seconds (Positive) and for 30 to 60 seconds is weak positive.

Observation

S. No	Characterization	Observation
1	Color of the filter paper	
2	Time to develop the color	

Report

Chapter 37

Phenylalanine Deaminase Test (PDA Test)

Object

1. To understand the biochemical basis of Phenylalanine Deaminase Test.
2. To perform Phenylalanine Deaminase Test.

Principle

The PDA test is performed to differentiate among the urea positive gram negative bacilli based on the ability to produce phenylpyruvic acid by oxidative deamination.

Phenylalanine is an amino acid that, upon deamination by the enzyme oxidase yields phenylpyruvic acid, which is detected by light to deep green cyclic compound by the chelating of α-keto acid with ferric chloride solution added to the medium.

Material Required

Culture: 24 hour cultures of *Proteus mirabilis* (Positive) and *E.coli.* (Negative).

Medium: Phenylalanine Agar Medium.

Table 37.1

S. No	Composition	Amount for 1000 mL
1	DL-Phenylalanine	2.0 gm
2	Yeast Extract	3.0 gm
3	Sodium Chloride	5.0 gm
4	Sodium Phosphate	1.0 gm
5	Agar	12.0 gm
6	Deionized Water	1000 mL
pH – 7.4 ± 0.2 at 25°C		

Autoclave at 121°C for 15 minutes.

Chemical Required

10% Ferric chloride Reagent acidified – dissolve 12.0 gm of ferric chloride in 97.5 mL of distill water and slowly add 2.5 mL of concentrated HCl.

Instrument Required

Inoculating loop and needle, autoclave, laminar airflow cabinet and incubator.

Procedure

1. Take the required quantity of Phenylalanine Agar slant and mark with the microorganism to be inoculated.
2. Inoculate the microorganism by streaking the slant in fishtail motion aseptically.
3. Incubate at 35 °C for 18 to 24hrs.
4. After incubation add 4 to 5 drops of ferric chloride solution.
5. Observe for the development of green color within 1 to 5 minutes.

Observation

S. No	Characterization	Observation
1	Color of the slant	

Report

Chapter 38

Starch Hydrolysis Test

Object

1. To understand the biochemical basis of Starch hydrolysis Test.
2. To perform Starch hydrolysis Test.

Principle

The Starch hydrolysis test is performed to identify the bacteria having ability to secrete amylase or endoamylase.

The bacteria which are having the ability to excrete amylase or endoamylase hydrolyze the amylose or starch to maltose and glucose. To the starch agar if iodine is added it develops blue color because of the reaction between iodine and helical structure of amylase, if the hydrolysis occurs leads to the breakdown of the structure and there is no color development.

Material Required

Culture: 24 hour cultures of *Streptococcus bovis* (Positive) and *Enterococcus faecalis* (Negative).

Medium: Mueller Hinton Agar Medium.

Table 38.1

S. No.	Composition	Amount for 1000 mL
1	Beef Extract	2.0 gm
2	Acid Hydrolysate of Casein	17.5 gm
3	Starch	1.5 gm
4	Agar	17.0 gm
5	Deionized Water	1000 mL
pH – 7.3 ± 0.1 at 25ºC		

Autoclave at 121ºC for 15 minutes.

Chemical Required

Grams Iodine, Mueller Hinton Agar Petri dish.

Instrument Required

Inoculating loop and needle, autoclave, laminar airflow cabinet and incubator.

Procedure

1. Inoculate the microorganism by streaking the petri dish in fishtail motion aseptically.
2. Incubate at 35°C for 48 to 72 hrs.
3. After incubation, flood with grams iodine dropwise.
4. Observe for halos around the colony.

Observation

S. No.	Characterization	Observation
1	Color of the media	
2	Color around the colony	

Report

Chapter 39

Urea Test

Object

1. To understand the biochemical basis of Urea Test.
2. To perform Urea Test.

Principle

This test is performed for the identification of several genera and species of *Enterobacteriaceae*, including *Proteus, Klebsiella, Yersinia, Citrobacter* and *Cornybacterium*.

This test identify the bacteria having ability to secrete enzyme urease which split the urea in the presence of water to release two molecules of ammonia and carbon dioxide. The ammonia combines with CO_2 and forms ammonium carbonate turns the medium alkaline, it is identified by the pH indicator phenol red turns the color from orange yellow to bright pink.

Material Required

Culture: 24 hour cultures of *Proteus mirabilis* (Positive) and *Escherichia coli* (Negative).

Medium: Christensen's Urea Agar Medium.

Table 39.1

S. No	Composition	Amount for 1000 mL
1	Gelatine peptone	1.0 gm
2	D(+)-Glucose	1.0 gm
3	Potassium dihydrogen phosphate	2.0 gm
4	Sodium chloride	5.0 gm
5	Phenol red	0.012 gm
6	Agar	12.0 gm
7	Deionized Water	950 mL
pH – 6.8 ± 0.2 at 25°C		

Autoclave at 121°C for 15 minutes and add 50 mL of sterile 40% Urea Solution when the temperature is reached 50°C after sterilization.

Chemical Required

Christensen's Urea Agar Slant.

Instrument Required

Inoculating loop and needle, autoclave, laminar airflow cabinet and incubator.

Procedure

1. Inoculate the microorganism by streaking the Slant in fishtail motion aseptically.
2. Incubate at 35°C to 37°C.
3. Observe the development of pink color as long as 7 days.

Observation

S. No.	Characterization	Observation
1	Color of the media	

Report

Chapter 40

Lipase Test

Object

1. To understand the biochemical basis of Lipase Test.
2. To perform Lipase Test.

Principle

This test identifies the bacteria having ability to secrete enzyme lipases which hydrolyze the breakdown of triglycerides into glycerol and free fatty acids. Fatty acids are insoluble and cause opacity to the media, producing the iridescent sheen on the colonies and surface of the media.

Material Required

Culture: 24 hour cultures of *Staphylococcus aureus* (Positive) and *Escherichia coli* (Negative).

Medium: Egg Yolk Agar Medium Modified.

Table 40.1

S. No	Composition	Amount for 1000 mL
1	Pancreatic Digest of Casein	15.0 gm
2	Papaic Digest of Soybean Meal	5.0 gm
3	Yeast Extract ...	5.0 gm
4	Sodium chloride	5.0 gm
5	L-Cystine	0.4 gm
6	Agar	20.0 gm
7	Hemin	5.0 mg
8	Egg Yolk Suspension	100 mL
9	Deionized Water	900 mL
pH – 6.8 ± 0.2 at 25°C		

Autoclave at 121°C for 15 minutes and adds 100 mL of Egg yolk suspension.

Chemical Required

Christensen's Urea Agar Slant.

Instrument Required

Inoculating loop and needle, autoclave, laminar airflow cabinet and incubator.

Procedure

1. Inoculate the microorganism by streaking the Slant in fishtail motion aseptically.
2. Incubate at 35 ℃ to 37 °C for 24 to 48hrs.
3. Observe the development of iridescent sheen (mother of pearl) on the surface of the colony and the surrounding agar.

Observation

S. No.	Characterization	Observation
1	Presence of iridescent sheen	

Report

Chapter 41

Lecithinases Test

Object

1. To understand the biochemical basis of Lecithinases Test.
2. To perform Lecithinases Test.

Principle

This test identifies the bacteria having ability to secrete enzyme lecithinases or phospholipases which split the lecithovitellin, a lipoprotein component of the egg yolk to form phosphoryl choline and insoluble diglyceride, which forms precipitate to the media, appears as a white opaque halo around the colony.

Material Required

Culture: 24 hour cultures of *Bacillus cereus* (Positive) and *Escherichia coli* (Negative).

Medium: Egg Yolk Agar Medium Modified.

S. No	Composition	Amount for 1000 mL
1	Pancreatic Digest of Casein	15.0 gm
2	Papaic Digest of Soybean Meal	5.0 gm
3	Yeast Extract ...	5.0 gm
4	Sodium chloride	5.0 gm
5	L-Cystine	0.4 gm
6	Agar	20.0 gm
7	Hemin	5.0 mg
8	Egg Yolk Suspension	100 mL
9	Deionized Water	900 mL
pH – 6.8 ± 0.2 at 25°C		

Autoclave at 121 °C for 15 minutes and adds 100 ml of Egg Yolk Suspension.

Chemical Required

Christensen's Urea Agar Slant.

Instrument Required

Inoculating loop and needle, autoclave, laminar airflow cabinet and incubator

Procedure

1. Inoculate the microorganism by streaking the slant in fishtail motion aseptically.
2. Incubate at 35 ºC to 37 °C for 24 to 48hrs.
3. Observe the development of milky white halo around the colony.

Observation

S. No.	Characterization	Observation
1	Presence of milky white halo	

Report

Chapter 42

Alkaline Phosphotase Test

Object

1. To understand the biochemical basis of Alkaline Phosphotase Test.

2. To perform Alkaline Phosphotase Test.

Principle

It is one of the rapid biochemical tests for the identification of anaerobes. This test used to differentiate between the indole positive species *Peptostreptococcus hydrogenalis* and *Peptostreptococcus asaccharolyticus*. The bacteria having the ability to release alkaline Phosphotase causes hydrolysis of 4-nitrophenyl phosphate to 4-nitro phenol, which is yellow in color.

Material Required

Culture: 24 hour cultures of Peptostreptococcus hydrogenalis (Positive) and Peptostreptococcus asaccharolyticus (Negative).

Chemical Required

Wee-Tab PO_4 (Alk.Phosphatase) Kit of Key Scientific products or from other companies containing p-Nitrophenol phosphate (alkaline phosphatase) (PO_4) as their ingredient.

The tablets contain approximately 0.05 mg of p-Nitrophenol phosphate in a Sodium Chloride and Dicalcium phosphate base.

Instrument Required

Inoculating loop and needle, autoclave, laminar airflow cabinet and incubator.

Procedure

1. Add 3-5 drops of this solution to the tube containing the tablet, shaking to disintegrate the tablet.
2. Inoculate heavily with a loopful of organism from a fresh pure 24 hour culture plate or slant. Mix with the loop until the organism is in suspension.
3. Incubate at 34 ºC to 37°C for 2 to 24 hrs.
4. Observe the development of yellow color, the Vortexing or shaking the test vigorously will enhance color development.

Observation

S. No.	Characterization	Observation
1	Color of the suspension	

Report

Chapter 43

Glutamic Acid Decarboxylase Test

Object

1. To understand the biochemical basis of Glutamic acid Decarboxylase Test.
2. To perform Glutamic acid Decarboxylase Test.

Principle

Glutamic acid Decarboxylase is the rapid biochemical tests for the identification of *Bacteroides fragilis, Clostridium perfringens, Clostridium sordellii, Clostridium baratii, Eubacterium limosum and Peptostreptococcus micros.*

The bacteria having the enzymatic ability to decarboxylate glutamic acid to an amine, which increases the pH in alkaline region.

Material Required

Culture: 24 hour cultures of *Bacteroides fragilis* (Positive) and *Fusobacterium nucleatum* (Negative).

Medium: Glutamic acid Decarboxylase Medium Modified.

S. No	Composition	Amount for 1000 mL
1	L-glutamic acid	2.0 gm
2	Bromcresol green-sodium salt	0.07 gm
3	Triton X-155	0.3 mL
4	Agar	3.0 gm
5	Distilled Water	1000 mL
pH – 6.8 ± 0.2 at 25ºC		

Autoclave at 121ºC for 15 minutes.

Instrument Required

Inoculating loop and needle, autoclave, laminar airflow cabinet and incubator.

Procedure

1. Stab the inoculum at several spots at the top of the medium and the macerate the upper part of the medium by moving the loop in and out of the medium several times.
2. Incubate aerobically at 35 ℃ to 37°C for 1 to 2 hrs.
3. Observe the color change of the medium from green to deep blue.

Observation

S. No.	Characterization	Observation
1	Color of the medium	

Report

Chapter 44

L- Alanyl- Alanylaminopeptidase Test

Object

1. To understand the biochemical basis of L-Alanyl- Alanylamino-peptidase Test.
2. To perform L- Alanyl- Alanylaminopeptidase Test.

Principle

L- Alanyl- Alanylaminopeptidase Test is the rapid biochemical tests to separate *Bacteroides* species *from Fuscobacterium* species.

The bacteria secreting the enzyme L- Alanyl- Alanylaminopeptidase causes hydrolysis of L- Alanyl- Alanylaminopeptide to beta-naphthylamine, which form complex with paradimethyl amino-cinnamaldehyde in presence of acetic acid to produce a pink to purple.

Material Required

Culture: 24 hour cultures of *Bacteroides fragilis* (Positive) and *Fusobacterium nucleatum* (Negative).

Chemical required: K9145B ALN disc from key scientific or similar disc. Cinnamaldehyde.

Instrument Required

Inoculating loop and needle, autoclave, laminar airflow cabinet and incubator.

Procedure

1. Place a disc onto a clean slide and moisten slightly.
2. Using a sterile stick or loop, smear the disc with a visible paste of the suspected isolate. False negatives may result from insufficient inoculum.

3. Incubate at room temperature for 5 minutes.

4. Add 1 drop of PEP reagent and wait 2 minutes to observe color from red to pink.

Observation

S. No.	Characterization	Observation
1	Color of the Disc	

Report

Chapter 45

L-Proline – Aminopeptidase Test

Object

1. To understand the biochemical basis of L-Proline – Aminopeptidase test (PRO).
2. To perform L-Proline – Aminopeptidase test.

Principle

L-Proline – Aminopeptidase test is the rapid biochemical test for the identification of *Clostridium difficile* in a selective media.

The bacteria secreting the enzyme L-Proline – Aminopeptidase test causes hydrolysis of L-Proline beta-naphthylamide to beta-naphthylamine, which form complex with paradimethyl aminocinnamaldehyde in presence of acetic acid to produce a pink to purple color.

Material Required

Culture: 24hour cultures of *Clostridium difficile* (Positive) and *Fusobacterium nucleatum* (Negative).

Chemical required: Hardy Diagnostics C. diff PROTM Test Kit. Cinnamaldehyde.

Principle of the Kit: Hardy Diagnostics C. diff PROTM Test Kit allows for rapid screening of PRO activity and indole production by suspected *C. difficile* isolates in a convenient and easy to use card format. The card contains Circle A for indole production identification, while Circle B is impregnated with a proline substrate for L-proline amino-peptidase for PRO identification. Following inoculation on the card, indole production and PRO activity are detected using the same color development reagent. *C. difficile* isolates should produce a negative (colorless to pink) result in Circle A (indole production) and a positive (dark blue to purple) result in Circle B (PRO activity). It is important to note that some bacterial species that are positive for indole production may also demonstrate a false positive result for PRO activity.

Instrument Required

Inoculating loop and needle, autoclave, laminar airflow cabinet and incubator.

Procedure

1. Moisten Circle A and Circle B with one drop of deionized water. Do not over saturate the test area.
2. Using a sterile loop or applicator stick, remove a heavy, visible paste of suspected *Clostridium difficile* (2-3 colonies) and smear onto Circle A. Repeat this step for Circle B.
3. Incubate the test card for 5 minutes at room temperature (15-30 °C.).
4. After incubation, add one drop of the cinnamaldehyde reagent to Circle A and Circle B.
5. Observe the color development of dark blue - purple for positives and negatives will take place within 30 seconds.

Observation

S. No.	Characterization	Observation
1	Color of the Disc	

Report

Chapter 46

Spot Indole Test

Object

1. To understand the biochemical basis of Spot Indole Test.
2. To perform Spot Indole Test.

Principle

Spot Indole Test is important for the identification of anerobic bacteria. The bacteria having the ability to produce the enzyme tryptophanase can split the Indole from tryptophan, it is identified by the formation of colored adduct complex by the reaction of indole with p-dimethyl-amminocinnamaldehyde.

Material Required

Culture: 24 hour cultures of *Escherichia coli* (Positive) and *Pseudomonas aeruginosa* (Negative).

Medium: Egg Yolk Agar Medium Modified.

S. No	Composition	Amount for 1000 mL
1	Pancreatic Digest of Casein	15.0 gm
2	Papaic Digest of Soybean Meal	5.0 gm
3	Yeast Extract	5.0 gm
4	Sodium chloride	5.0 gm
5	L-Tryptophan	0.2 gm
6	L-Cystine	0.4 gm
7	Agar	20.0 gm
8	Hemin	5.0 mg
9	Egg Yolk Suspension	100 mL
10	Deionized Water	900 mL
pH – 6.8 ± 0.2 at 25ºC		

Autoclave at 121 ºC for 15 minutes and adds 100ml of Egg Yolk Suspension.

Chemical required: p-dimethyl- amminocinnamaldehyde reagent is prepared by dissolving 1 gm of p-dimethyl- amminocinnamaldehyde in 100 mL of 10%v/v HCl.

Instrument Required

Inoculating loop and needle, autoclave, laminar airflow cabinet and incubator.

Procedure

1. The microorganism is inoculated in Egg Yolk Agar medium containing the tryptophan and incubated at 35°C to 37°C for 24 to 48hrs.
2. A piece of Whatman filter paper No 1 is placed in a Petri disc cover and the paper was moistened with the reagent (paper should be saturated and not wet).
3. Remove the colonies from the media with the help of the loop and rub on the filter paper.
4. Observe the development of blue or green color on the filter paper around the inoculum in 30 seconds.

Observation

S. No.	Characterization	Observation
1	Color of the filter paper around the inoculum	

Report

Chapter 47

Bile Test

Object

1. To understand the biochemical basis of Bile Test.
2. To perform Bile Test.

Principle

Bile Test is important for the differentiation of anaerobic gram negative rods. *Bacteroides fragilis, Fusobacterium mortiferum* and *Fusobacterium varium* has the ability to grow in presence of 20% bile or 2% oxgall.

Material Required

Culture: 24 hour cultures of *Bacteroides fragilis* (Positive) and *Pseudomonas melaninogenica* (Negative).

Chemical required: The filter paper disks impregnated with 25 mg of oxgall (Difco) or Bile disks were prepared with a thick solution containing 1 g of oxgall (Difco) per mL of distilled water. The solution was sterilized at 121ºC for 15 min and then delivered to sterile, dry filter paper disks (Schleicher & Schuell no. 740-E), using a 25μL Oxford pipette.

Instrument Required

Inoculating loop and needle, autoclave, laminar airflow cabinet and incubator.

Procedure

1. Fresh culture of the test organism in thioglycollate broth is streaked on to a Brucella Blood Agar Plate in three directions to obtain a heavy, confluent growth.
2. Aseptically place a Bile Disk onto the agar surface.

3. Incubate the blood agar plate anaerobically at 35°C for up to 48 hours.

4. Observe the Growth up to the edge of the disk (<16-mm) for resistance (Positive result).

Observation

S. No.	Characterization	Observation
1	Growth of the inoculum	

Report

PART - V

Chapter 48

Bacterial Growth Curve Analysis and its Environmental Applications

Object

Bacteria are among the most abundant life forms on Earth. They are found in every ecosystem and are vital for everyday life. For example, bacteria affect what people eat, drink, and breathe, and there are actually more bacterial cells within a person's body than mammalian cells. Because of the importance of bacteria, it is preferable to study particular species of bacteria in the laboratory. To do this, bacteria are grown under controlled conditions in pure culture, meaning that only one type of bacterium is under consideration. Bacteria grow quickly in pure culture, and cell numbers increase dramatically in a short period of time. By measuring the rate of cell population increase over time, a "growth curve" to be developed. This is important when aiming to utilize or inoculate known numbers of the bacterial isolate, for example to enhance plant growth, increase biodegradation of toxic organics, or produce antibiotics or other natural products at an industrial scale.

Principles

Bacterial reproduction occurs via binary fission, in which one bacterial cell divides and becomes two cells (**Figure 48.1**). The time needed for cell division is known as the mean generation time, or doubling time, which is the time needed for the number of cells to double.

Each cell division results in a doubling of the cell number. At low cell numbers, the increase is not very large; however after a few generations, cell numbers increase explosively. After n divisions, there are 2^n cells.

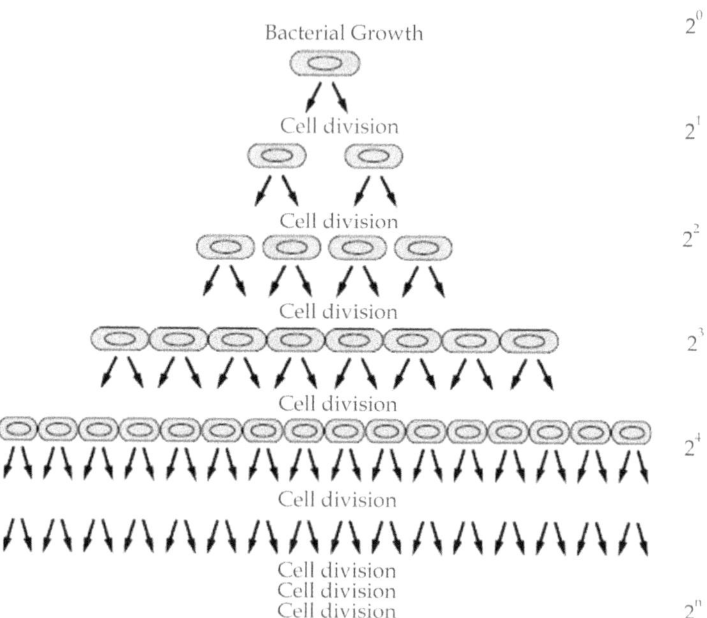

Fig. 48.1 Exponential cell division.

To understand and define the growth of particular microorganisms, they are placed in a flask, where the nutrient supply and environmental conditions are controlled. If the liquid medium supplies all the nutrients required for growth and environmental parameters conducive to growth, the increase in numbers can be measured as a function of time to obtain a growth curve. Several distinct growth phases can be observed within a growth curve (**Figure 48.2**). These include the lag phase, the exponential or log phase, the stationary phase, and the death phase, each of which are associated with specific physiological changes (**Table 48.1**).

Table 48.1 The four phases of bacterial growth.

Phase	Characteristics
Lag Phase	Slow growth or lack of growth due to physiological adaptation of cells to culture conditions or dilution of exoenzymes due to initial low cell densities.
Exponential or Log Phase	Optimal growth rates, during which cell numbers double at discrete time intervals known as the mean generation time.
Stationary Phase	Growth (cell division) and death of cells counterbalance each other resulting in no net increase in cell numbers. The reduced growth rate is usually due to a lack of nutrients and/or a buildup of toxic waste constituents.
Death Phase	Death rate exceeds growth rate resulting in a net loss of viable cells.

Overall, it is often critical to determine bacterial growth kinetics for a given bacterial isolate, in order to know the number of bacterial cells present in the liquid medium. There are different ways to measure growth in a liquid medium, including turbidity measurements using a colorimetric spectrophotometer, and serial dilution plating. Turbidity measurements rely on the fact that the more cells present in the liquid medium, the more turbid the liquid becomes. Serial dilution plating involves assaying the number of cells in the liquid medium that can form viable colonies on solid culture, a measurement known as the culture's "colony-forming units". Note, however, that such plating assays can only be used for bacteria that are, in fact, culturable.

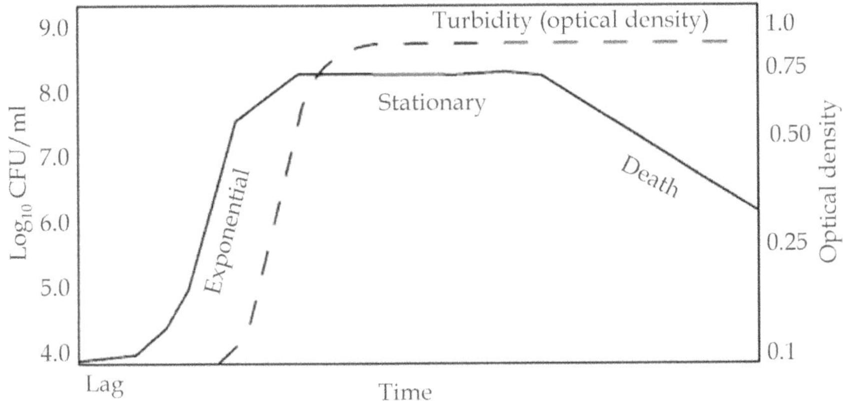

Fig. 48.2 A typical growth curve for a bacterial population.

Compare the shape of the curves based on colony-forming units (CFUs) versus optical density, particularly in the death phase. The difference is due to the fact that dead cells still result in turbidity, but cannot form viable colonies in culture.

Procedure

1. Collection of Bacterial Culture Aliquots

(a) One day before collection of growth time points, inoculate 20 mL of trypticase soy broth (TSB) medium in a 50-mL flask with *E. coli*.

(b) Incubate overnight at 27 °C. This relatively long incubation period results in a stationary phase population of wild type *E. coli* of approximately 10^9 CFU/mL.

(c) On the following day, use 100 µL of the prepared culture to inoculate 250 mL of TSB (in a 500-mL flask). Mix thoroughly.

Remove a 5-mL aliquot and refrigerate immediately at 4 °C. This is T = 0 or T_0 time point, and should contain approximately 4 x 10^5 CFU/mL.

(d) Place the flask of the remaining *E. coli* (245 mL) in a 37 °C shaking incubator. Remove 5-mL aliquots of culture every hour, up to 8 h. Store each aliquot at 4 °C. Designate these aliquots T_1 through T_8.

2. Serial Dilution

(a) Remove aliquots of *E. coli* from the refrigerator and place on ice for transporting. Keep all cultures on ice until use.

(b) Set up a series of dilution tubes to obtain various dilutions of each *E. coli* culture (**Figure 48.3**). Microfuge tubes are convenient for this function. Each dilution tube should have 900 µL of dilution fluid (sterile saline). A dilution series is needed for each *E. coli* culture (T_0 through T_8); label each tube according to **Table 48.2**.

(c) Begin dilutions by adding 100 µL of *E. coli* from the tube labeled T_0 (the initial *E. coli* culture) to tube A, which is the 10^{-1} dilution of T_0. Vortex the tube for 5 s.

(d) Subsequently, add 100 µL of Tube A to the next tube of saline, Tube B, which is the 10^{-2} dilution of T_0. Continue the needed dilution series for each time point aliquot. Remember to vortex each tube prior to transfer. It is also important to use a new pipette tip for each transfer.

Table 48.2 Labeling of series of dilution tubes

E. coli culture	Dilutions needed and Tube #						
	A	**B**	**C**	**D**	**E**	**F**	**G**
T_0	10^{-1}	10^{-2}					
T_1	10^{-1}	10^{-2}					
T_2	10^{-1}	10^{-2}	10^{-3}				
T_3	10^{-1}	10^{-2}	10^{-3}	10^{-4}			
T_4	10^{-1}	10^{-2}	10^{-3}	10^{-4}	10^{-5}		
T_5	10^{-1}	10^{-2}	10^{-3}	10^{-4}	10^{-5}	10^{-6}	
T_6	10^{-1}	10^{-2}	10^{-3}	10^{-4}	10^{-5}	10^{-6}	10^{-7}
T_7	10^{-1}	10^{-2}	10^{-3}	10^{-4}	10^{-5}	10^{-6}	
T_8	10^{-1}	10^{-2}	10^{-3}	10^{-4}	10^{-5}	10^{-6}	

Dilution series required for each *E. coli* culture.

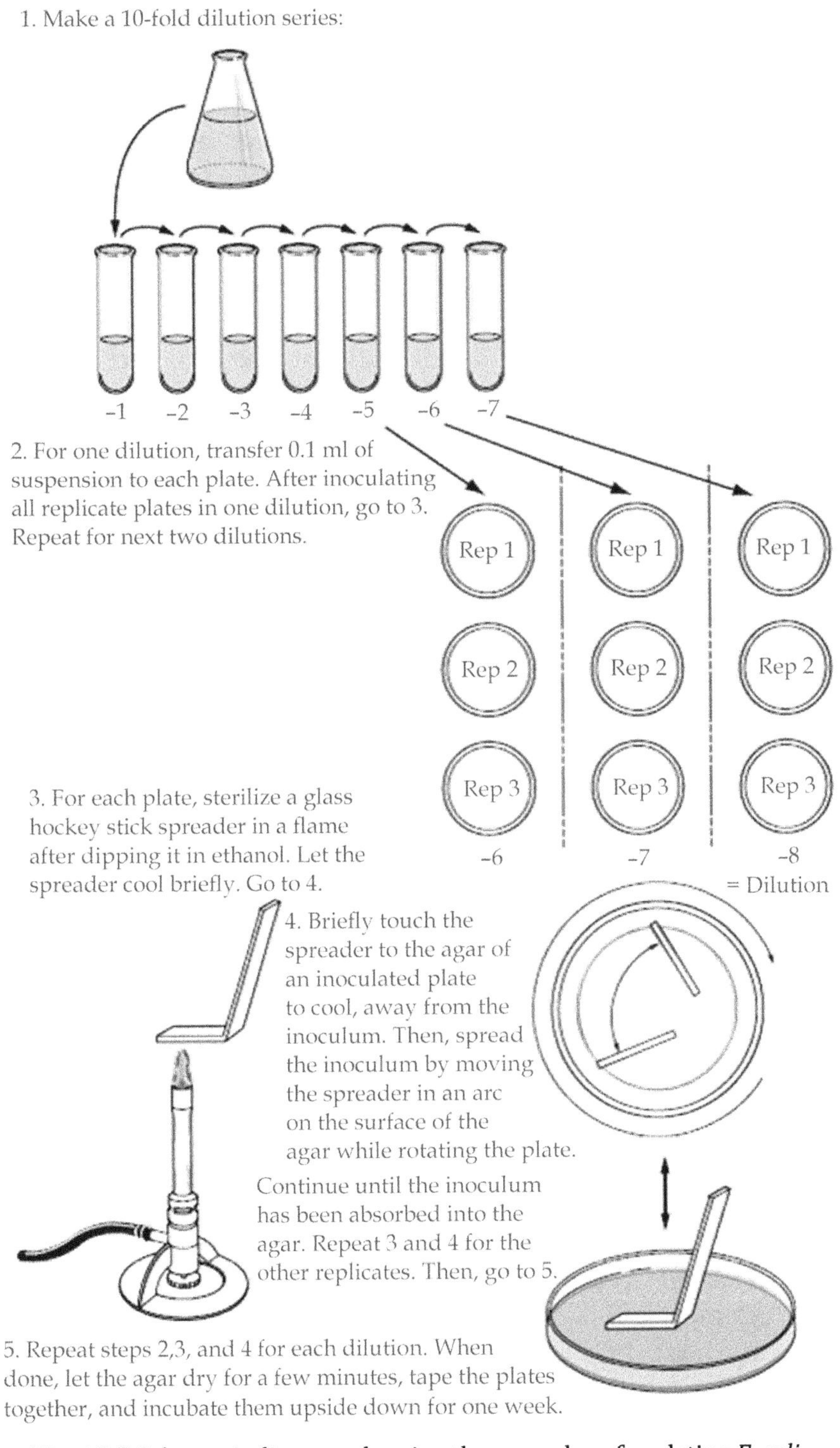
1. Make a 10-fold dilution series:
-1 -2 -3 -4 -5 -6 -7
2. For one dilution, transfer 0.1 ml of suspension to each plate. After inoculating all replicate plates in one dilution, go to 3. Repeat for next two dilutions.
Rep 1
Rep 2
Rep 3
-6
-7
-8
= Dilution
3. For each plate, sterilize a glass hockey stick spreader in a flame after dipping it in ethanol. Let the spreader cool briefly. Go to 4.
4. Briefly touch the spreader to the agar of an inoculated plate to cool, away from the inoculum. Then, spread the inoculum by moving the spreader in an arc on the surface of the agar while rotating the plate.
Continue until the inoculum has been absorbed into the agar. Repeat 3 and 4 for the other replicates. Then, go to 5.
5. Repeat steps 2,3, and 4 for each dilution. When done, let the agar dry for a few minutes, tape the plates together, and incubate them upside down for one week.

Fig. 48.3 Schematic diagram showing the procedure for plating *E. coli.*

3. Plating

(a) Three dilutions for each *E. coli* culture time point aliquot will be plated, according to **Table 48.3**. Label plates with the time point (T_1 through T_8), the dilution factor, and volume to be added. Use triplicate plates for each dilution.

(b) Add 100 μL of each dilution to the plate by pipetting the amount to the center of the agar plate (**Figure 48.3**). Immediately spread the aliquot by utilizing a flame sterilized "L" shaped glass rod. If the aliquot is not spread immediately, it sorbs *in situ* on the plate, resulting in bacterial overgrowth at the spot of initial inoculation.

(c) Repeat the plating for each dilution series for time points T_1 through T_8. Remember to sterilize the rod between plates and especially between different dilutions.

(d) Once plates have dried for a few minutes, invert and place in 37°C incubator overnight. Inverting the plates preclude condensation from falling onto the agar plate. Following overnight incubation, plates should be stored in refrigerator.

Table 48.3 Dilutions of *E. coli* Culture Time Point Aliquot

E.coli culture	Dilutions to be plated		
T_0	10^{-1}	10^{-2}	10^{-3}
T_1	10^{-1}	10^{-2}	10^{-3}
T_2	10^{-2}	10^{-3}	10^{-4}
T_3	10^{-3}	10^{-4}	10^{-5}
T_4	10^{-4}	10^{-5}	10^{-6}
T_5	10^{-5}	10^{-6}	10^{-7}
T_6	10^{-6}	10^{-7}	10^{-8}
T_{7*}	10^{-5}	10^{-6}	10^{-7}
T_{8*}	10^{-4}	10^{-5}	10^{-6}

*Lower dilutions take into account lower populations due to death phase.

Plating protocol for *E. coli* cultures.

4. Counting Colonies and Calculating Mean Generation Time

(a) Examine plates for uniformity of colonies and lack of contamination.

(b) For each time point (T_0 through T_8), pick one dilution that contains between 30 and 300 colonies, and count triplicate plates.

(c) Using the dilution factor, back-calculate the number of cells per mL of original culture at time points T_0 through T_8. For example, if the number of colonies resulting from a 10^{-4} dilution is 30, 28, and 32: Mean number of colonies = 30 colonies

These arose from 0.1 mL of a 10^{-4} dilution

Number of colonies per mL = $30 \times 10^4 = 3 \times 10^6$

(d) Plot $\log_{10}$ CFU/mL versus time (in hours).

(e) From the graph, identify the exponential phase of growth. Using 2 time points within the exponential growth phase and the corresponding cell numbers at each time, calculate the mean generation time.

Results

Following a serial dilution plating experiment, the following data was obtained. At the beginning of exponential growth designated here as time t = 0, the initial concentration of bacterial cells is 1,000 CFU/mL. At time t = 6 h, the concentration of cells is 16,000 CFU/mL.

Now, $X = 2^n \times X_0$

Where:

X_0 = initial concentration of cells = 1,000 CFU/mL

X = concentration of cells after time t = 16,000 CFU/mL

n = number of generations

16,000 = $2^n \times 1,000$

$2^n = 16$

$\log_{10} 2^n = \log_{10} 16$

$n \times 0.301 = 1.204$

$$n = \frac{1.204}{0.301} = 4$$

Four generations elapsed in 6 h, so

Mean Generation Time = 6/4 = 1.5 h.

Applications and Summary

Knowledge of bacterial growth kinetics and bacterial numbers in a culture medium is important from both a research and commercial point of view. In research, it is often critical to know the number of bacteria in a sample, so the experiment can be replicated, if need be, with the exact same numbers. For example, during experiments in which bacterial inoculants are added to a plot of soil, a minimum of 10^4 CFU needs to be added per gram of soil to get the desired effect, such as enhanced biodegradation of toxic organic soil contaminants. Another example is the case of commercially produced rhizobial inoculants, where known numbers of rhizobia (bacteria that enter into symbiotic relationships with the roots of plants) are impregnated into a peat-based carbon medium. The medium is then used to inoculate legume seeds to enhance biological nitrogen fixation (*i.e.*, the conversion of molecular nitrogen into organic forms that can be used by organisms as nutrients).

Growth kinetics is also useful for assessing whether particular strains of bacteria are adapted to metabolize certain substrates, such as industrial waste or oil pollution. Bacteria that are genetically engineered to clean up oil spills, for example, can be grown in the presence of complex hydrocarbons to ensure that their growth would not be repressed by the toxic effects of oil. Similarly, the slope and shape of growth curves produced from bacteria grown with mixtures of industrial waste products can inform scientists whether the bacteria can metabolize the particular substance, and how many potential energy sources for the bacteria can be found in the waste mixture.

PART - VI

Chapter 49

Determination of Phenol Coefficient

Phenol coefficient of a disinfectant is calculated by dividing the dilution of test disinfectant by the dilution of phenol that disinfects under predetermined conditions.

Rideal Walker Method

Phenol is diluted from 1:400 to 1:800 and the test disinfectant is diluted from 1:95 to 1:115. Their bactericidal activity is determined against Salmonella typhi suspension. Subcultures are performed from both the test and phenol at intervals of 2.5, 5, 7.5 and 10 minutes. The plates are incubated for 48-72 hours at 37°C. That dilution of disinfectant which disinfects the suspension in a given time is divided by that dilution of phenol which disinfects the suspension in same time gives its phenol coefficient.

Disinfectant	Dilution	Growth of test organism in subculture after exposure for:			
		2.5 mins	5 mins	7.5 mins	10 mins
Test disinfectant	1:400	NG	NG	NG	NG
	1:500	G	NG	NG	NG
	1:600	G	G	NG	NG
	1:700	G	G	G	NG
	1:800	G	G	G	G
Phenol	1:95	G	NG	NG	NG
	1:100	G	G	NG	NG
	1:105	G	G	G	NG
	1:110	G	G	G	NG
	1:115	G	G	G	G

For example, after 7.5 minutes, the test organism was killed by the test disinfectant at a dilution of 1;600. In the same period the test organism was killed by phenol at a dilution of 1:100.

Phenol Coefficient=600/100=6

This result indicates that the test disinfectant can be diluted six times as much as phenol and still possess equivalent killing power for the test organism.

Disadvantages of the Rideal-Walker test are

No organic matter is included; the microorganism Salmonella typhi may not be appropriate; the time allowed for disinfection is short; it should be used to evaluate phenolic type disinfectants only.

Chick Martin test

This test also determines the phenol coefficient of the test disinfectant. Unlike in Rideal Walker method where the test is carried out in water, the disinfectants are made to act in the presence of yeast suspension (or 3% dried human feces) to simulate the presence or organic matter. Time for subculture is fixed at 30 minutes and the organism used to test efficacy is S.typhi as well as S.aureus. The phenol coefficient is lower than that given by Rideal Walker method.

	Rideal -Walker	**Chick-Martin**
Volume medium	5.0 mL	10.0 mL
Diluent for test disinfectant	Distilled water	Water with yeast suspension or feces
Reaction temperature	17.5±0.5ºC	30º±0.5ºC
Organism	Salmonella typhi	Salmonella typhi, Staphylococcus aureus
Sampling times	2.5, 5.0, 7.5, 10.0 min	30.0 min
Calculation of coefficient	Dilution test killing in 7.5 mins divided by same for phenol	Mean concentration of phenol showing no growth after 30 min. divided by same for test

The phenol coefficient test recommended by AOAC included two test organisms (S. aureus and P. aeruginosa) and included the disinfectant inactivators in the recovery medium. The recovery medium Letheen broth contains the inactivator Lecithin and Polysorbate 80. In separate tests, the bacterial suspensions are added to standard dilutions of pure phenol and several dilutions of the test disinfectant. After contact time of 5, 10 and 15 minutes, samples are transferred to the recovery medium by a standard wire loop. When the positive and negative cultures have been recorded, the result of the test is expressed as phenol coefficient. It is calculated by dividing the highest dilution of the disinfectant that kills the test inoculum in ten minutes but not in five minutes by the dilution of phenol that gives the same result.

Disinfectant Kill Time Test

This test was designed to demonstrate log reduction values over time for a disinfectant against selected bacteria, fungi, and/or mold. The most common organisms tested include: Bacillus subtilis, Bacillus atrophaeus, Bacillus thuringiensis, Staphylococcus aureus, Salmonella cholerasuis, Pseudomonas aeruginosa, Aspergillus niger, and Trichophyton mentagrophytes. A tube of disinfectant is placed into a waterbath for temperature control and allowed to equilibrate. Once the tube has reached temperature, it is inoculated to achieve a concentration of approximately 106 CFU/mL. At selected time points (generally five points are used including zero) aliquots are removed and placed into a neutralizer blank. Dilutions of the neutralizer are made and selected dilutions plated onto agar. Colonies are enumerated and log reductions are calculated.

Capacity Tests

Each time a soiled instrument is placed into a container with disinfectant, a certain quantity of dirt and bacteria is added to the solution. The ability to retain activity in the presence of an increasing load is the capacity of the disinfectant. In a capacity test, the disinfectant is challenged repeatedly by successive additions of bacterial suspension until its capacity to kill has been exhausted. Capacity tests simulate the practical situations of housekeeping and instrument disinfection. The best known capacity test is the Kelsey-Sykes test.

Kelsey-Sykes test is a triple challenge test, designed to determine concentrations of disinfectant that will be effective in clean and dirty conditions. The disinfectant is challenged by three successive additions of a bacterial suspension during the course of the test. The duration of test takes over 30 minutes to perform. The concentration of the disinfectant is reduced by half by the addition of organic matter (autoclaved yeast cells), which builds up to a final concentration of 0.5%. Depending on the type of disinfectant, a single test organism is selected from S. aureus, P. aeruginosa, P. vulgaris and E. coli. The method can be carried out under 'clean' or 'dirty' conditions. The dilutions of the disinfectant are made in hard water for clean conditions and in yeast suspension for dirty conditions. Test organism alone or with yeast is added at 0, 10 and 20 minutes interval. The contact time of disinfectant and test organism is 8 min.

The three sets of five replicate cultures corresponding to each challenge are incubated at 32 ºC for 48 hours and growth is assessed by turbidity. The disinfectant is evaluated on its ability to kill microorganisms or lack of it and the result is reported as a pass or a fail and not as a coefficient. Sets that contain two or more negative cultures are recorded as a negative result. The disinfectant passes at the dilution tested if negative results are obtained after the first and second challenges. The third challenge is not included in the pass/fail criterion but positive cultures serve as inbuilt controls. If there are no positive cultures after the third challenge, a lower concentration of the disinfectant may be tested.

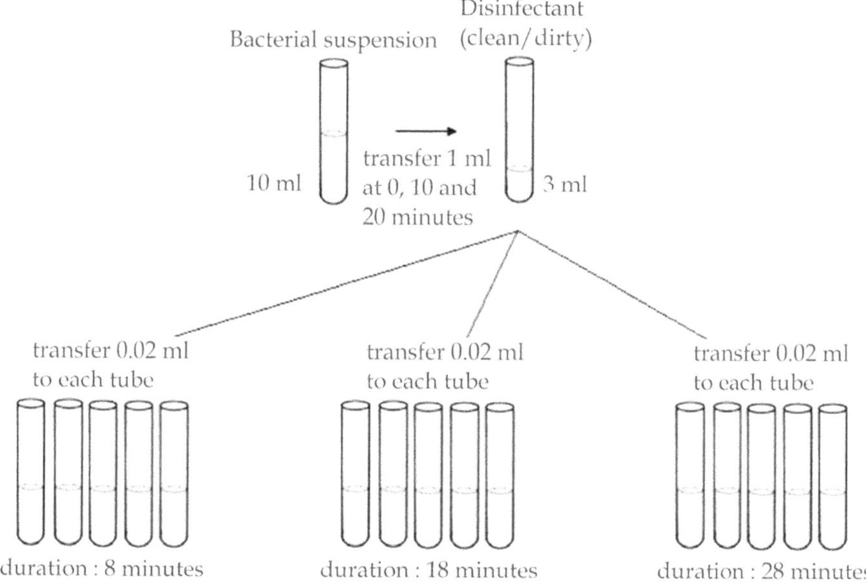

Fig. 49.1 Determination of phenol coefficient.

Specimen Result of a Test

Concentration	Inoculum count	Challenge number			Result
		1	2	3	
1.0	2×10^9	+++++	+++++	+++++	Fail
1.5	2×10^9	- - - - +	- - +++	+++++	Pass
2.0	2×10^9	- - - - -	- - - - -	- - - - +	Pass

The capacity test of Kelsey and Sykes gives a good guideline for the dilution of the preparation to be used. Disadvantage of this test is the fact that it is rather complicated.

Test for Stability and Long-term Effectiveness

Recommended concentrations based on Kelsey Sykes test apply only to freshly prepared solutions but if the solutions are likely to be kept for more than 24 hours, the effectiveness of these concentrations must be confirmed by a supplementary test for stability of unused solution and for the ability of freshly prepared and stale solutions to prevent multiplication of a small number of bacteria that may have survived the short term exposure. *P. aeruginosa* is used a test organism. Sufficient disinfectant solution is prepared for two tests. One portion is inoculated immediately and tested for growth after holding for seven days at room temperature. The other portion is kept at room temperature for seven days and then inoculated with a freshly prepared suspension of test organism. It is also tested for growth seven days after inoculation. If growth is detected, a higher concentration of disinfectant must be tested in the same way.

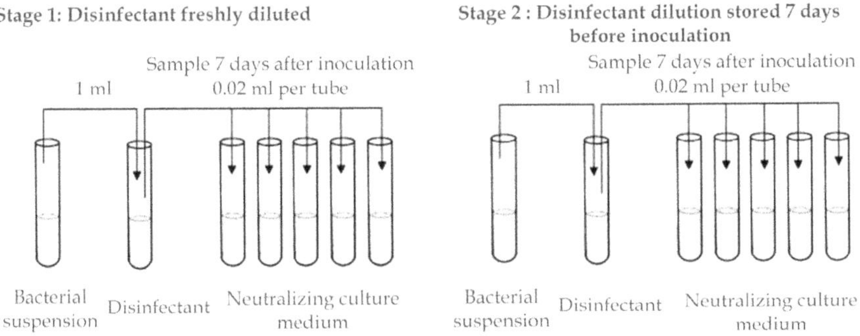

Fig. 49.2 Test for stability and long-term effectiveness.

Practical Tests

The practical tests under real-life conditions are performed after measuring the time-concentration relationship of the disinfectant in a quantitative suspension test. The objective is to verify whether the proposed use dilution is still adequate in the conditions under which it would be used. The best known practical tests are the surface disinfection tests. Surface tests assess the effectiveness of the selected sanitizer against surface-adhered microorganisms. The test surface (a small tile, a microscopic slide, a piece of PVC, a stainless steel disc, etc.) is contaminated with a standardized inoculum of the test bacteria and dried; then a definite volume of the disinfectant solution is distributed over the carrier; after the given exposure time the number of survivors is determined by impression on a contact plate or by a rinsing technique, in which the carrier is rinsed in a diluent, and the number of bacteria is determined in the rinsing fluid. In order to determine the spontaneous dying rate of the organisms caused by drying on the carrier, a control series is included in which the disinfectant is substituted by distilled water; from the comparison of the survivors in this control series with the test series, the reduction is determined quantitatively.

There is an essential difference between a carrier test and a surface disinfectant test: in the former case the carrier is submerged in the disinfectant solution during the whole exposure time, whereas in the latter case the disinfectant is applied on the carrier for the application time and thereafter the carrier continues to dry during the exposure. Surface tests can reflect in-use conditions like contact times, temperatures, use-dilutions, and surface properties.

Surface Time Kill Test

A 24 hour culture in nutrient broth culture is prepared. A volume of microbial culture (usually 0.010 mL to 0.020 mL) is placed onto the center of each of a number of sterile test surfaces. This inoculum can be spread over the sterile test surface in a circular pattern to achieve a thin, uniform coverage with the test microorganism if desired. To measure initial microbial concentrations, one or more untreated, inoculated test surfaces are harvested and microorganisms are enumerated. The remaining inoculated test surfaces are treated with the disinfectant, each for a different length of time. Immediately after the treatment times have elapsed, the test surfaces are placed into a solution that neutralizes the disinfecting action of the product, and microorganisms surviving treatment with the disinfectant or sanitizer are cultured and enumerated. Results of the timekill study are tabulated and reported, usually by charting microbial concentrations on the test surfaces as a function of treatment time with the disinfectant or sanitizer.

In-use Test

A simple to use test was described by Maurer in 1985 that can be used in hospitals and laboratories to detect contamination of disinfectants. A 1 mL sample of the disinfectant is added to 9 mL diluent which also contains an inactivator. Ten drops, each of 0.02 mL volume of the diluted sample are placed on each of two nutrient agar plates. One is incubated at 37 ºC for three days and the other at room temperature for seven days. Five or more colonies on either plate indicate contamination.

British Standard Tests for Quaternary Ammonium Compounds

This test was initially described in 1960 to distinguish bactericidal action from the high level of bacteriostatic activity, which is characteristic of QACs. This test is also applicable to other bactericides such as chlorhexidine and synthetic phenols. The inactivator used contains 2% lecithin and 3% non-ionic detergent (polysorbate 80). The test is performed using suspensions of gram negative and gram positive bacteria with or without the inclusion of organic matter. If a series of samples are taken from a dilution of the disinfectant containing 5×108 to 5×109 bacteria per mL at the start of the test, a death curve may be prepared from the colony counts on the agar containing recovery medium and reduction factors up to 106 (99.99% kill) can be verified. In order to determine the antimicrobial value of QAC, it was revised as the highest dilution of the disinfectant that, under the test conditions, will reduce the microbial population to a colony count not greater than 0.01% of that in the control. In this revision, E. coli was used and the contact time was 10 minutes. The challenge medium is E. coli culture suspension with equal amount of horse serum. One mL of the challenge is added to nine mL of each dilution of the disinfectant along with two control tubes containing diluent alone. At the end of exposure period, one mL each of the mixture is added to 9 mL of inactivator and the surviving bacteria are counted as colony forming units on agar plates.

Testing Schemes

The antimicrobial efficiency of a disinfectant is examined at three stages of testing. The first phase concerns laboratory tests in which it is verified whether a chemical compound or a preparation possesses antimicrobial activity: for these preliminary screening tests essentially quantitative suspension tests are considered. The second stage is still carried out in the laboratory but in conditions simulating real-life conditions. Not disinfectants, but disinfection procedures are examined. It is determined in the practical tests in which conditions and at which use-dilution after a given contact time the preparation is active. The third phase comprises the field tests or pilot studies, and the variant of in-use tests. In these tests it is verified whether, after a normal period of use, germs in the disinfectant solution are still killed.

Most studied are the bactericidal tests in which the activity towards vegetative bacteria is examined. AOAC has schedules that are applicable for fungi and yeasts too (fungicidal tests), for mycobacteria (tuberculocidal tests), for viruses (virucidal tests) and for spores of bacteria (sporicidal tests).

Bactericidal tests

A bactericidal test must include the following sequence of steps:
1. The test organism is exposed to a suitable concentration of the disinfectant.
2. Samples are taken at specified times and added immediately to a diluent or culture medium containing the appropriate disinfectant inactivator.
3. The treated samples are cultured for surviving microorganisms.

Test Organisms

Specified strains (usually ATCC) of *S. aureus, P. aeruginosa, P. vulgaris* and *E. coli* are usually recommended. A synthetic broth is recommended for preparing a series of subcultures to be used in the tests. The 24-hour broth culture may be used without further treatment; however, it is usually filtered (to remove slime) and centrifuged. The washed bacteria are resuspended in hard water to which autoclaved yeast or serum may be added to simulate dirty conditions. Finally, the suspension is shaken with glass beads on a vortex mixer and a viable count is set up immediately before performing the test.

The Disinfectant

The concentration or dilution of the disinfectant to be tested may be based on manufacturer's recommendations. The solutions should be prepared on the day of test. Distilled water or standard hard water is used to make dilutions. Tap water is unsuitable because it may contain chemicals that may precipitate with some disinfectants.

PART - VII

Chapter 50

Test for Sterility

The test is applied to substances or preparations which, according to the Pharmacopoeia, are required to be sterile. However, a satisfactory result only indicates that no contaminating microorganism has been found in the sample examined in the conditions of the test.

Precautions Against Microbial Contamination

The test for sterility is carried out under aseptic conditions. In order to achieve such conditions, the test environment has to be adapted to the way in which the sterility test is performed. The precautions taken to avoid contamination are such that they do not affect any microorganisms which are to be revealed in the test. The working conditions in which the tests are performed are monitored regularly by appropriate sampling of the working area and by carrying out appropriate controls.

Culture Media and Incubation Temperatures

Media for the test may be prepared as described below, or equivalent commercial media may be used provided that they comply with the growth promotion test.

The following culture media have been found to be suitable for the test for sterility. Fluid thioglycollate medium is primarily intended for the culture of anaerobic bacteria; however, it will also detect aerobic bacteria. Soya-bean casein digest medium is suitable for the culture of both fungi and aerobic bacteria.

Fluid Thioglycollate Medium

L-Cystine	0.5 g
Agar	0.75 g
Sodium chloride	2.5 g
Glucose monohydrate/anhydrous	5.5/5.0 g

Table *Contd....*

Yeast extract (water-soluble)	5.0 g
Pancreatic digest of casein	15.0 g
Sodium thioglycollate or	0.5 g
Thioglycollic acid	0.3 mL
Resazurin sodium solution (1 g/l of resazurin sodium), freshly prepared	1.0 mL
Water R	1000 mL
pH after sterilization 6.9 to 7.3.	

Mix the L-cystine, agar, sodium chloride, glucose, water-soluble yeast extract and pancreatic digest of casein with the water R and heat until solution is effected. Dissolve the sodium thioglycollate or thioglycollic acid in the solution and, if necessary, add sodium hydroxide (1 mol/L) VS so that, after sterilization, the solution will have a pH of 9 to 7.3. If filtration is necessary heat the solution again without boiling and filter while hot through moistened filter paper. Add the resazurin sodium solution, mix and place the medium in suitable vessels which provide a ratio of surface to depth of medium such that not more than the upper half of the medium has undergone a colour change indicative of oxygen uptake at the end of the incubation period. Sterilize using a validated process. If the medium is stored, store at a temperature between 2°C and 25°C in a sterile, airtight container. If more than the upper one-third of the medium has acquired a pink colour, the medium may be restored once by heating the containers in a water-bath or in free-flowing steam until the pink colour disappears and cooling quickly, taking care to prevent the introduction of non-sterile air into the container. Do not use the medium for a longer storage period than has been validated.

Fluid thioglycollate medium is to be incubated at 30–35 °C.

F or products containing a mercurial preservative that cannot be tested by the membrane-filtration method, fluid thioglycollate medium incubated at 20–25 °C may be used instead of soya-bean casein digest medium provided that it has been validated as described in growth promotion test.

Alternative Thioglycollate Medium

Where prescribed or justified and authorized, the following alternative thioglycollate medium might be used. Prepare a mixture having the same composition as that of the fluid thioglycollate medium, but omitting the agar and the resazurin sodium solution, sterilize as directed above. The pH after sterilization is 6.9 to 7.3. Heat in a water-bath prior to use and incubate at 30–35 °C under anaerobic conditions.

Soya-bean casein digest medium

Pancreatic digest of casein	17.0 g
Papaic digest of soya-bean meal	3.0 g
Sodium chloride	5.0 g
Dipotassium hydrogen phosphate	2.5 g
Glucose monohydrate/anhydrous	2.5/2.3 g
Water R	1000 mL
pH after sterilization 7.1 to 7.5.	

Dissolve the solids in water R, warming slightly to effect solution. Cool the solution to room temperature. Add sodium hydroxide (1 mol/L) VS, if necessary, so that after sterilization the solution will have a pH of 7.1 to 7.5. Filter, if necessary, to clarify, distribute into suitable vessels and sterilize using a validated process. Store at a temperature between 2 °C and 25 °C in a sterile well-closed container, unless it is intended for immediate use. Do not use the medium for a longer storage period than has been validated.

Soya-bean casein digest medium is to be incubated at 20–25 °C.

The media used comply with the following tests, carried out before or in parallel with the test on the product to be examined.

***Sterility*:** Incubate portions of the media for 14 days. No growth of microorganisms occurs.

***Growth promotion test of aerobes, anaerobes and fungi*:** Test each batch of ready-prepared medium and each batch of medium prepared either from dehydrated medium or from ingredients. Suitable strains of microorganisms are indicated in Table 50.1.

Inoculate portions of fluid thioglycollate medium with a small number (not more than 100 CFU) of the following microorganisms, using a separate portion of medium for each of the following species of microorganism: *Clostridium sporogenes, Pseudomonas aeruginosa, Staphylococcus aureus*. Inoculate portions of soya-bean casein digest medium with a small number (not more than 100 CFU) of the following microorganisms, using a separate portion of medium for each of the following species of microorganism: *Aspergillus brasiliensis, Bacillus subtilis, Candida albicans*. Incubate for not more than 3 days in the case of bacteria and not more than 5 days in the case of fungi.

Seed-lot culture maintenance techniques (seed-lot systems) are used so that the viable microorganisms used for inoculation are not more than five passages removed from the original master seed-lot.

The media are suitable if a clearly visible growth of the microorganisms occurs.

Table 50.1 Strains of the test microorganisms suitable for use in the Growth promotion test and the Method suitability test

Aerobic bacteria	
Staphylococcus aureus	ATCC 6538, CIP 4.83, NCTC 10788, NCIMB 9518, NBRC 13276
Bacillus subtilis	ATCC 6633, CIP 52.62, NCIMB 8054, NBRC 3134
Pseudomonas aeruginosa	ATCC 9027, NCIMB 8626, CIP 82.118, NBRC 13275
Anaerobic bacterium	
Clostridium sporogenes	ATCC 19404, CIP 79.3, NCTC 532 *or* ATCC 11437, NBRC 14293
Fungi	
Candida albicans	ATCC 10231, IP 48.72, NCPF 3179, NBRC 1594
Aspergillus brasiliensis	ATCC 16404, IP 1431.83, IMI 149007, NBRC 9455

Method Suitability Test

Carry out a test as described below under Test for sterility of the product to be examined using exactly the same methods except for the following modifications.

Membrane filtration: After transferring the content of the container or containers to be tested to the membrane add an inoculum of a small number of viable microorganisms (not more than 100 CFU) to the final portion of sterile diluent used to rinse the filter.

Direct inoculation: After transferring the contents of the container or containers to be tested to the culture medium add an inoculum of a small number of viable microorganisms (not more than 100 CFU) to the medium.

In both cases use the same microorganisms as those described above under Growth promotion test of aerobes, anaerobes and fungi. Perform a growth promotion test as a positive control. Incubate all the containers containing medium for not more than 5 days.

If clearly visible growth of microorganisms is obtained after the incubation, visually comparable to that in the control vessel without product, either the product possesses no antimicrobial activity under the conditions of the test or such activity has been satisfactorily eliminated. The test for sterility may then be carried out without further modification.

If clearly visible growth is not obtained in the presence of the product to be tested, visually comparable to that in the control vessels without product, the product possesses antimicrobial activity that has not been satisfactorily eliminated under the conditions of the test. Modify the conditions in order to eliminate the antimicrobial activity and repeat the method suitability test.

This method suitability is performed:

(a) When the test for sterility has to be carried out on a new product;

(b) Whenever there is a change in the experimental conditions of the test.

The method suitability may be performed simultaneously with the Test for sterility of the product to be examined.

Test for Sterility of the Product to be Examined

The test may be carried out using the technique of membrane filtration or by direct inoculation of the culture media with the product to be examined. Appropriate negative controls are included. The technique of membrane filtration is used whenever the nature of the product permits, that is, for filterable aqueous preparations, for alcoholic or oily preparations and for preparations miscible with or soluble in aqueous or oily solvents provided these solvents do not have an antimicrobial effect in the conditions of the test.

Membrane filtration: Use membrane filters having a nominal pore size not greater than 0.45 µm whose effectiveness to retain microorganisms has been established. Cellulose nitrate filters, for example, are used for aqueous, oily and weakly alcoholic solutions and cellulose acetate filters, for example, for strongly alcoholic solutions. Specially adapted filters may be needed for certain products, e.g. for antibiotics.

The technique described below assumes that membranes about 50 mm in diameter will be used. If filters of a different diameter are used the volumes of the dilutions and the washings should be adjusted accordingly. The filtration apparatus and membrane are sterilized by appropriate means. The apparatus is designed so that the solution to be examined can be introduced and filtered under aseptic conditions; it permits the aseptic removal of the membrane for transfer to the medium or it is suitable for carrying out the incubation after adding the medium to the apparatus itself.

Aqueous solutions: If appropriate, transfer a small quantity of a suitable, sterile diluent such as a 1 g/L neutral solution of meat or casein peptone pH 6.9 to 7.3 onto the membrane in the apparatus and filter. The diluent may contain suitable neutralising substances and/or appropriate inactivating substances for example in the case of antibiotics.

Transfer the contents of the container or containers to be tested to the membrane or membranes, if necessary after diluting to the volume used in the method suitability test with the chosen sterile diluent but in any case using not less than the quantities of the product to be examined prescribed in Table 50.2. Filter immediately. If the product has antimicrobial properties, wash the membrane not less than three times by filtering through it each time the volume of the chosen sterile diluent used in the method suitability test. Do not exceed a washing cycle of five times 100 mL per filter, even if during method suitability it has been demonstrated that such a cycle does not fully eliminate the antimicrobial activity. Transfer the whole membrane to the culture medium or cut it aseptically into two equal parts and transfer one half to each of two suitable media. Use the same volume of each medium as in the method suitability test. Alternatively, transfer the medium onto the membrane in the apparatus. Incubate the media for not less than 14 days.

Table 50.2 Minimum quantity to be used for each medium

Quantity per container	Minimum quantity to be used for each medium unless otherwise justified and authorized
Liquids	
• Less than 1 mL	The whole contents of each container
• 1-40 mL	Half the contents of each container but not less than 1 mL
• Greater than 40 mL and not greater than 100 mL	20 mL
• Greater than 100 mL	10 per cent of the contents of the container but not less than 20 mL
Antibiotic liquids	1 mL
Insoluble preparations, creams and ointments to be suspended or emulsified	Use the contents of each container to provide not less than 200 mg
Solids	
• Less than 50 mg	The whole contents of each container
• 50 mg or more but less than 300 mg	Half the contents of each container but not less than 50 mg
• 300 mg – 5 g	150 mg
• Greater than 5 g	500

Soluble solids: Use for each medium not less than the quantity prescribed in Table 50.2 of the product dissolved in a suitable solvent such as the solvent provided with the preparation, water for injections R, sodium chloride (9 g/L) TS or peptone (1 g/L) TS1 and proceed with the test as described above for aqueous solutions using a membrane appropriate to the chosen solvent.

Oils and oily solutions: Use for each medium not less than the quantity of the product prescribed in Table 50.2. Oils and oily solutions of sufficiently low viscosity may be filtered without dilution through a dry membrane. Viscous oils may be diluted as necessary with a suitable sterile diluent such as isopropyl myristate R shown not to have antimicrobial activity in the conditions of the test. Allow the oil to penetrate the membrane by its own weight then filter, applying the pressure or suction gradually. Wash the membrane at least three times by filtering through it each time about 100 mL of a suitable sterile solution such as peptone (1 g/L) TS1 containing a suitable emulsifying agent at a concentration shown to be appropriate in the method suitability test, for example polysorbate 80 at a concentration of 10 g/L. Transfer the membrane or membranes to the culture medium or media or vice versa as described above for aqueous solutions, and incubate at the same temperatures and for the same times.

Ointments and creams: Use for each medium not less than the quantities of the product prescribed in Table 50.2. Ointments in a fatty base and emulsions of the water-in-oil type may be diluted to 1 per cent in isopropyl myristate R as described above, by heating, if necessary, to not more than 40 °C. In exceptional cases it may be necessary to heat to not more than 44 °C. Filter as rapidly as possible and proceed as described above for oils and oily solutions.

Direct inoculation of the culture medium: Transfer the quantity of the preparation to be examined prescribed in Table 50.2 directly into the culture medium so that the volume of the product is not more than 10% of the volume of the medium, unless otherwise prescribed.

If the product to be examined has antimicrobial activity, carry out the test after neutralizing this with a suitable neutralizing substance or by dilution in a sufficient quantity of culture medium. When it is necessary to use a large volume of the product it may be preferable to use a concentrated culture medium prepared in such a way that it takes account of the subsequent dilution. Where appropriate the concentrated medium may be added directly to the product in its container.

Oily liquids: Use media to which have been added a suitable emulsifying agent at a concentration shown to be appropriate in the method suitability of the test, for example polysorbate 80 at a concentration of 10 g/L.

Ointments and creams: Prepare by diluting to about 1 in 10 by emulsifying with the chosen emulsifying agent in a suitable sterile diluent such as peptone (1 g/L) TS1. Transfer the diluted product to a medium not containing an emulsifying agent.

Incubate the inoculated media for not less than 14 days. Observe the cultures several times during the incubation period. Shake cultures containing oily products gently each day. However, when fluid thioglycollate medium is used for the detection of anaerobic microorganisms keep shaking or mixing to a minimum in order to maintain anaerobic conditions.

Observation and Interpretation of Results

At intervals during the incubation period and at its conclusion, examine the media for macroscopic evidence of microbial growth. If the material being tested renders the medium turbid so that the presence or absence of microbial growth cannot be readily determined by visual examination, 14 days after the beginning of incubation transfer portions (each not less than 1 ml) of the medium to fresh vessels of the same medium and then incubate the original and transfer vessels for not less than 4 days.

If no evidence of microbial growth is found, the product to be examined complies with the test for sterility. If evidence of microbial growth is found the product to be examined does not comply with the test for sterility, unless it can be clearly demonstrated that the test was invalid for causes unrelated to the product to be examined. The test may be considered invalid only if one or more of the following conditions are fulfilled:

(a) The data of the microbiological monitoring of the sterility testing facility show a fault;

(b) A review of the testing procedure used during the test in question reveals a fault;

(c) Microbial growth is found in the negative controls;

(d) After determination of the identity of the microorganisms isolated from the test, the growth of this species or these species may be ascribed unequivocally to faults with respect to the material and/or the technique used in conducting the sterility test procedure.

If the test is declared to be invalid it is repeated with the same number of units as in the original test.

If no evidence of microbial growth is found in the repeat test the product examined complies with the test for sterility. If microbial growth is found in the repeat test the product examined does not comply with the test for sterility.

Application of the Test to Parenteral Preparations, Ophthalmic and Other Non-Injectable Preparations Required to Comply with the Test for Sterility

When using the technique of membrane filtration, use, whenever possible, the whole contents of the container, but not less than the quantities indicated in Table 50.2 diluting where necessary to about 100 mL with a suitable sterile solution, such as peptone (1 g/L) TS1.

When using the technique of direct inoculation of media, use the quantities shown in Table 50.2, unless otherwise justified and authorized. The tests for bacterial and fungal sterility are carried out on the same sample of the product to be examined. When the volume or the quantity in a single container is insufficient to carry out the tests, the contents of two or more containers are used to inoculate the different media.

Minimum Number of Items to be Tested

The minimum number of items to be tested in relation to the size of the batch is given in Table 50.3.

Table 50.3 Minimum number of Items to be tested

Number of items in the batch*	Minimum number of items to be tested for each medium, unless otherwise justified and authorized**
Parenteral preparations	
Not more than 100 containers	10 percent or 4 containers whichever is the greater
More than 100 but not more than 500 containers	10 containers
More than 500 containers	2 percent or 20 containers (10 containers for large-volume parenterals) whichever is the less
Ophthalmic and other non-injectable preparation	
Not more than 200 containers	5 percent or 2 containers whichever is the greater
More than 200 containers	10 containers
If the product is presented in the form of single-dose containers, apply the scheme shown above for preparations for parenteral use	

Table 50.3 Contd....

Number of items in the batch*	Minimum number of items to be tested for each medium, unless otherwise justified and authorized**
Bulk solid products	
Up to 4 containers	Each container
More than 4 containers but not more than 50 containers	20 percent or 4 containers whichever is the greater
More than 50 containers	2 percent or 10 containers whichever is the greater

*If the batch size is not known, use the maximum number of items prescribed

**If the contents of one container are enough to inoculate the two media, this column gives the number of containers needed for both the media together.

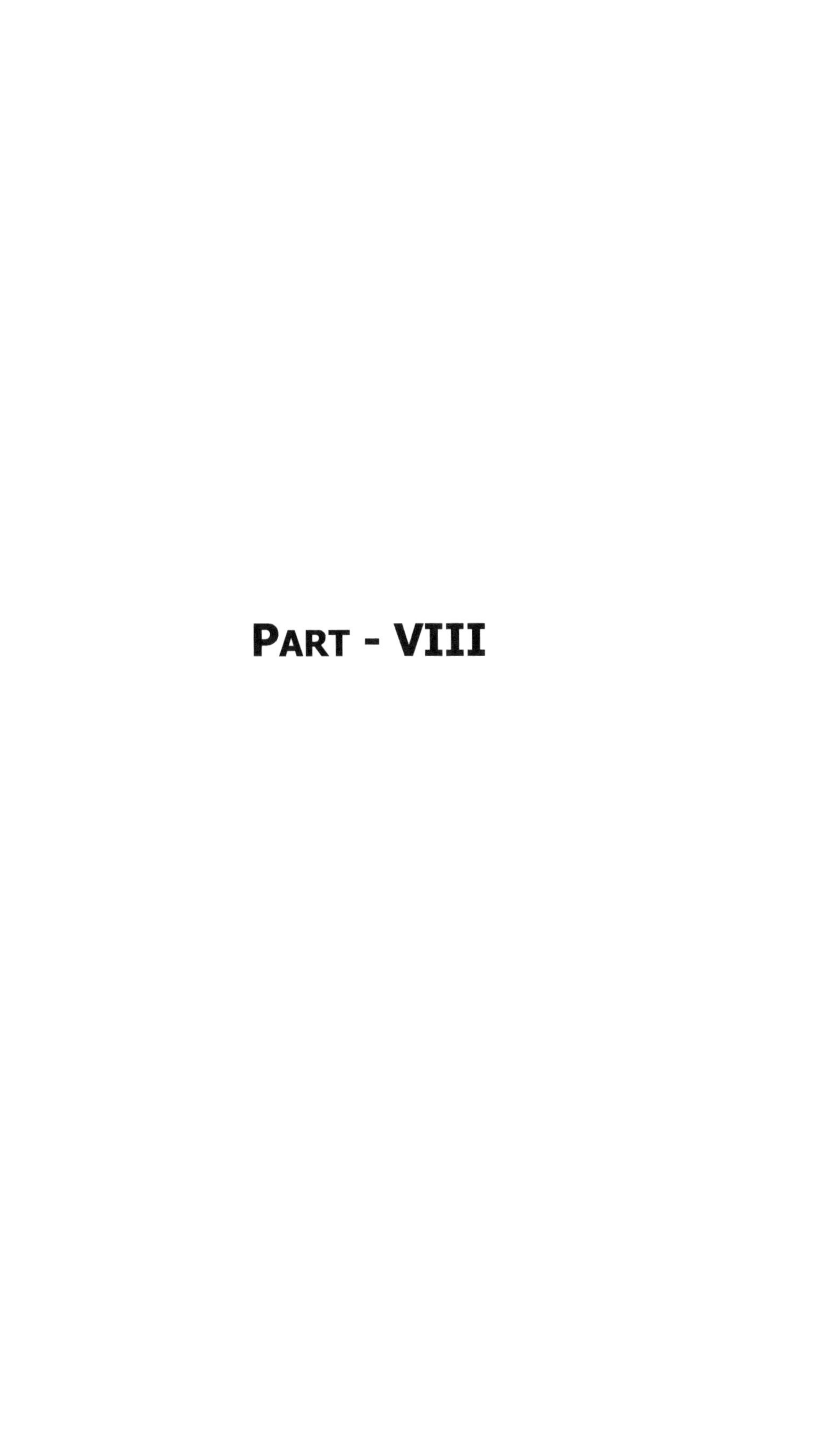

Part - VIII

Chapter 51

Microbial Assay of Antibiotics

Introduction and General Information

The activity (potency) of antibiotics can be demonstrated by their inhibitory effect on microorganisms under suitable conditions. A reduction in antimicrobial activity may not be adequately demonstrated by chemical methods. This chapter summarizes procedures for the antibiotics recognized in the United States Pharmacopeia (USP) for which the microbiological assay is the standard analytical method.

Two general techniques are employed: the cylinder-plate (or plate) assay and the turbidimetric (or tube) assay.

Table 51.1 Lists of all the antibiotics that contain microbial assays and specifies the type of assay (cylinder-plate or turbidimetric).

Antibiotic	Type of Assay
Amphotericin B	Cylinder-plate
Bacitracin	Cylinder-plate
Bleomycin	Cylinder-plate
Capreomycin	Turbidimetric
Carbenicillin	Cylinder-plate
Chloramphenicol	Turbidimetric
Chlortetracycline	Turbidimetric
Cloxacillin	Cylinder-plate
Colistemethate	Cylinder-plate
Colistin	Cylinder-plate
Dihydrostreptomycin	Cylinder-plate
	Turbidimetric
Erythromycin	Cylinder-plate
Gentamicin	Cylinder-plate
Gramicidin	Turbidimetric
Nafcillin	Cylinder-plate

Table 51.1 *Contd...*

Antibiotic	Type of Assay
Natamycin	Cylinder-plate
Neomycin	Cylinder-plate
	Turbidimetric
Novobiocin	Cylinder-plate
Nystatin	Cylinder-plate
Oxytetracycline	Turbidimetric
Paromomycin	Cylinder-plate
Penicillin G	Cylinder-plate
Polymyxin B	Cylinder-plate
Sisomicin	Cylinder-plate
Tetracycline	Turbidimetric
Thiostrepton	Turbidimetric
Troleandomycin	Turbidimetric
Tylosin	Turbidimetric
Vancomycin	Cylinder-plate

[Note—Perform all procedures under conditions designed to avoid extrinsic microbial contamination. Take adequate safety precautions while performing these assays because of possible allergies to drugs and because live cultures of organisms are used in the procedures.]

Cylinder-plate assay: The cylinder-plate assay depends on diffusion of the antibiotic from a vertical cylinder through a solidified agar layer in a Petri dish or plate. The growth of the specific microorganisms inoculated into the agar is prevented in a circular area or zone around the cylinder containing the solution of the antibiotic.

Turbidimetric assay: The turbidimetric assay depends on the inhibition of growth of a microorganism in a uniform solution of the antibiotic in a fluid medium that is favorable to the growth of the microorganism in the absence of the antibiotic.

Units and Reference Standards: The potency of antibiotics is designated in either units (U) or µg of activity. In each case the unit or µg of antibiotic activity was originally established against a United States Federal Master Standard for that antibiotic. The corresponding USP Reference Standard is calibrated in terms of the master standard.

Originally, an antibiotic selected as a reference standard was thought to consist entirely of a single chemical entity and was therefore assigned a potency of 1000 µg/mg. In several such instances, as the manufacturing and purification methods for particular antibiotics became more advanced, antibiotics containing more than 1000 µg of activity/mg became possible. Such antibiotics had an activity equivalent to a given number of µg of the original reference standard. In most instances, however, the µg of activity is exactly equivalent numerically to the µg (weight) of the pure substance. In some cases, such as those listed below, the µg of activity defined in terms of the original master standard is equal to a unit:

1. Where an antibiotic exists as the free base and in salt form and the µg of activity has been defined in terms of one of these forms
2. Where the antibiotic substance consists of a number of components that are chemically similar but differ in antibiotic activity
3. Where the potencies of a family of antibiotics are expressed in terms of a reference standard consisting of a single member which, however, might itself be heterogeneous

Do not assume that the µg of activity corresponds to the µg (weight) of the antibiotic substance.

Apparatus: Labware used for the storage and transfer of test dilutions and microorganisms must be sterile and free of interfering residues. Use a validated sterilization method, such as dry heat, steam, or radiation; or use sterile, disposable labware.

Temperature control: Thermostatic control is required in several stages of a microbial assay: when culturing a microorganism and preparing its inoculum, and during incubation in plate and tube assays. Refer to specific temperature requirements below for each type of assay.

Test organisms: The test organism for each antibiotic is listed in Table 51.3 for the cylinder-plate assay and Table 51.8 for the turbidimetric assay. The test organisms are specified by the American Type Culture Collection (ATCC) number.

In order to ensure acceptable performance of test organisms, store and maintain them properly. Establish the specific storage conditions during method validation or verification. Discard cultures if a change in the organism's characteristics is observed.

Prolonged storage: For prolonged storage, maintain test organisms in a suitable storage solution such as 50% fetal calf serum in broth, 10%–15% glycerol in tryptic soy broth, defribinated sheep blood, or skim milk. Prolonged-storage cultures are best stored in the freeze-dried state; temperatures of – 60 ºC or below are preferred; temperatures below – 20 ºC are acceptable.

Primary cultures: Prepare primary cultures by transferring test organisms from prolonged-storage vials onto appropriate media, and incubate under appropriate growth conditions. Store primary cultures at the appropriate temperature, usually 2 ºC – 8 ºC, and discard after three weeks. A single primary culture can be used to prepare working cultures only for as many as seven days.

Working cultures: Prepare working cultures by transferring the primary culture onto appropriate solid media to obtain isolated colonies. Incubate working cultures under appropriate conditions to obtain satisfactory growth for preparation of test inocula. Prepare fresh working cultures for each test day.

Uncharacteristic growth or performance of a test organism: Use new stock cultures, primary cultures, or working cultures when a test organism shows uncharacteristic growth or performance.

Assay designs: Suitable experimental designs are key to increasing precision and minimizing bias. Control of the incubation parameters, temperature distribution and time, is critical for minimizing bias; it can be accomplished by staging the plates and racks as described for each assay.

Cylinder-plate assay: The comparisons are restricted to relationships between zone diameter measurements within plates, excluding the variation between plates. Individual plate responses are normalized on the basis of the relative zone size of the standard compared to the mean zone size of the standard across all plates.

Turbidimetric assay: To avoid systematic bias, place replicate tubes randomly in separate racks so that each rack contains one complete set of treatments. The purpose of this configuration is to minimize the influence of temperature distribution on the replicate samples. The turbidimetric assay, because of the configuration of the samples in test tube racks, is sensitive to slight variations in temperature. The influence of temperature variation can also be decreased by ensuring proper airflow or heat convection during incubation. At least three tubes for each sample and standard concentration (one complete set of samples) should be placed in a single rack. The comparisons are restricted to relationships between the observed turbidities within racks.

Potency considerations: Within the restrictions listed above, the recommended assay design employs a five-concentration standard curve and a single concentration of each sample preparation.

For the cylinder-plate assay, each plate includes only two treatments, the reference treatment (median level standard, i.e., S3) and one of the other four concentrations of the standard (S1, S2, S4, and S5) or the sample (U3). The concentration of the sample is an estimate based on the target concentration. The sample should be diluted to give a nominal concentration that is estimated to be equivalent to the median reference concentration (S3) of the standard. The purpose of diluting to the median reference concentration is to ensure that the sample result will fall within the linear portion of the standard curve. The test determines the relative potency of U3 against the standard curve. The sample (U3) should have a relative potency of about 100%. The final potency of the sample is obtained by multiplying the U3 result by the dilution factor.

An assay should be considered preliminary if the computed potency value of the sample is less than 80% or more than 125%. In this case, the results suggest that the sample concentration assumed during preparation of the sample stock solution was not correct. In such a case, one can adjust the assumed potency of the sample on the basis of the preliminary potency value and repeat the assay. Otherwise, the potency will be derived from a portion of the curve where the standard and sample responses will likely not be parallel.

Microbial determinations of potency are subject to inter-assay as well as intra-assay variables; therefore two or more independent assays are required for a reliable estimate of the potency of a given sample. Starting with separately prepared stock solutions and test dilutions of both the standard and the sample, perform additional assays of a given sample on a different day. The mean potency should include the results from all the valid independent assays. The number of assays required in order to achieve a reliable estimate of potency depends on the variability of the assay and the required maximum uncertainty for the potency estimate. The latter is assessed by the width of the confidence interval (refer to Calculations, Confidence limits and combinations of assay calculations). The combined result of a series of smaller, independent assays spread over a number of days is a more reliable estimate of potency than one from a single large assay with the same total number of plates or tubes. Note that additional assays or lower variability allows the product to meet tighter specification ranges. Reducing assay variability achieves the required confidence limit with fewer assays.

Cylinder-Plate Method

Temperature control: Use appropriately qualified and calibrated equipment to obtain the temperature ranges specified in Table 51.3.

Apparatus

Plates: Glass or disposable plastic Petri dishes (approximately 20 × 100 mm or other appropriate dimensions) with lids

Cylinders: Stainless steel or porcelain cylinders; 8 ± 0.1-mm o.d.; 6 ± 0.1-mm i.d.; 10 ± 0.1-mm high. [Note—Carefully clean cylinders to remove all residues; occasional cleaning in an acid bath, e.g., with about 2N nitric acid or with chromic acid is required.

Standard solutions: To prepare a stock solution, dissolve a suitable quantity of the USP Reference Standard of a given antibiotic, or the entire contents of a vial of USP Reference Standard, where appropriate, in the solvent specified in Table 51.2; and dilute to the specified concentration. Store at 2º–8 º, and use within the period indicated. On the day of the assay, prepare from the stock solution five or more test dilutions, in which the successive solutions increase stepwise in concentration, usually in the ratio of 1:1.25. Use the final diluent specified such that the median has the concentration suggested in Table 51.2.

Sample solutions: Assign an assumed potency per unit weight or volume to the sample. On the day of the assay prepare a stock solution in the same manner specified for the USP Reference Standard (Table 51.2). Dilute the sample stock solution in the specified final diluent to obtain a nominal concentration equal to the median concentration of the standard (S3).

Table 51.2 Sample solutions

| Antibiotic | Stock Solution | | | | | Test Dilution | |
	Initial Solvent	Initial Concen-tration	Further Diluent	Final Concentration	Use Within	Final Diluent	Median Concentration (S_3)[a,b]
Amphotericin B[c,d]	Dimethyl sulfoxide	—	—	1 mg/mL	Same day	B.10[e]	1 µg/mL
Bacitracin[f]	0.01 N hydrochloric acid	—	—	100 U/mL	Same day	B.1[e]	1 U/mL
Bleomycin	B.16[e]	—	—	2 U/mL	14 days	B.16[e]	0.04 U/mL
Carbenicillin	B.1[e]	—	—	1 mg/mL	14 days	B.1[e]	20 µg/mL

Table 51.2 *Contd...*

| Antibiotic | Stock Solution | | | | | Test Dilution | |
	Initial Solvent	Initial Concentration	Further Diluent	Final Concentration	Use Within	Final Diluent	Median Concentration (S_3)[a,b]
Cloxacillin	B.1[e]	—	—	1 mg/mL	7 days	B.1[e]	5 µg/mL
Colistemethate[c]	Water	10 mg/mL	B.6[e]	1 mg/mL	Same day	B.6[e]	1 µg/mL
Colistin	Water	10 mg/mL	B.6[e]	1 mg/mL	14 days	B.6[e]	1 µg/mL
Dihydrostreptomycin[g]	B.3[e]	—	—	1 mg/mL	30 days	B.3[e]	1 µg/mL
Erythromycin	Methanol	10 mg/mL	B.3[e]	1 mg/mL	14 days	B.3[e]	1 µg/mL
Gentamicin	B.3[e]	—	—	1 mg/mL	30 days	B.3[e]	0.1 µg/mL
Nafcillin	B.1[e]	—	—	1 mg/mL	2 days	B.1[e]	2 µg/mL
Natamycin	Dimethyl sulfoxide	—	—	1 mg/mL	Same day	B.10[e]	5 µg/mL
Neomycin[g]	B.3[e]	—	—	1 mg/mL	14 days	B.3[e]	1 µg/mL
Novobiocin	alcohol	10 mg/mL	B.3[e]	1 mg/mL	5 days	B.6[e]	0.5 µg/mL
Nystatin[c, h]	Dimethylformamide	—	—	1000 U/mL	Same day	B.6[e]	20 U/mL
Paromomycin	B.3[e]	—	—	1 mg/mL	21 days	B.3[e]	1 µg/mL
Penicillin G	B.1[e]	—	—	1000 U/mL	4 days	B.1[e]	1 U/mL
Polymyxin B[i]	Water	—	B.6[e]	10,000 U/mL	14 days	B.6[e]	10 U/mL
Sisomicin	B.3[e]	—	—	1 mg/mL	14 days	B.3[e]	0.1 µg/mL
Vancomycin	Water	—	—	1 mg/mL	7 days	B.4[e]	10 µg/mL

It is acceptable to adjust the median concentration to optimize zone sizes if the data remain in the linear range.

µg in this column refers to µg of activity.

Prepare the USP Reference Standard and sample test dilutions simultaneously.

Further dilute the stock solution with dimethyl sulfoxide to give concentrations of 12.8, 16, 20, 25, and 31.2 µg/mL before making the test dilutions. The test dilution of the sample should contain the same amount of dimethyl sulfoxide as the test dilutions of the USP Reference Standard.

The letter B refers to buffer. See Media and Solutions, Buffers for a description of each buffer listed in this table.

Each of the standard test dilutions should contain the same amount of hydrochloric acid as the test dilution of the sample.

The turbidimetric assay can be used as an alternative procedure.

Further dilute the stock solution with dimethylformamide to give concentrations of 256, 320, 400, 500, and 624 U/mL before making the test dilutions. Prepare the standard test dilutions simultaneously with test dilutions of the sample to be tested. The test dilution of the sample should contain the same amount of dimethylformamide as the test dilutions of the standard. Use low-actinic glassware.

Prepare the stock solution by adding 2 mL of water for each 5 mg of the USP Reference Standard.

Inocula: Suspend the test organism from a freshly grown slant or culture in 3 mL of sterile saline TS. Glass beads can be used to facilitate the suspension. Spread the saline suspension onto the surface of two or more agar plates (covering the entire surface) or onto the surface of a Roux bottle containing 250 mL of the specified medium (see Table 51.3).

Incubate for the specified time and at the temperature as specified in Table 51.3, or until growth is apparent.

After incubation, harvest the organism from the plates or Roux bottle with approximately 50 mL of sterile saline TS (except use Medium 34 for bleomycin; see the section Media and Solutions), using a sterile bent glass rod or sterile glass beads. Pipet the suspension into a sterile glass container. This is the harvest suspension.

Dilute an appropriate amount of the harvest suspension with sterile saline TS. Using the UV-visible spectrophotometer, measure % transmittance at 580 nm. The target value is approximately 25% transmittance at 580 nm. This value is used to standardize the harvest suspension volume added to the seed layer agar.

Starting with the suggested volumes indicated in Table 51.3, determine during method verification the proportions of stock suspension to be added to the inoculum medium that result in satisfactory zones of inhibition of approximately 14–16 mm in diameter for the median concentration of the standard (S3). [Note— Zone sizes that are outside the 11 to 19-mm range are not desirable, because these contribute to assay variability.] If the dilution percentage transmittance is above 25%, a ratio may be used to normalize the addition of organism to the seed layer. The normalization factor can be determined by dividing the percentage transmittance obtained from the dilution by 25. This ratio can then be multiplied by the suggested inoculum amount to obtain the volume (mL) of harvest suspension that needs to be added to the seed layer. Adjust the quantity of inoculum on a daily basis, if necessary, to obtain an optimum concentration–response relationship.

Alternatively, determine during method verification the proportion of harvest suspension to be incorporated into the inoculum, starting with the volumes indicated in Table 51.3, that result in satisfactory demarcation of the zones of inhibition of about 14–16 mm in diameter for the median concentration of the standard (S3) and giving a reproducible concentration–response relationship. Prepare the inoculum by adding a portion of stock suspension to a sufficient amount of agar medium that has been melted and cooled to 45°–50°.

Swirl the mixture without creating bubbles in order to obtain a homogeneous suspension.

Table 51.3 Inoculum of test organism in media

Antibiotic	Test Organism	ATCC[a] Number	Incubation Conditions			Suggested Inoculum Composition	
			Medium[b]	Temperature (°)	Time	Medium[b]	Amount (mL/100 mL)
Amphotericin B	Saccharomyces cerevisiae	9763	19	29–31	48 h	19	1.0
Bacitracin	Micrococcus luteus	10240	1	32–35	24 h	1	0.3
Bleomycin	Mycobacterium smegmatis	607	36	36–37.5	48 h	35	1.0
Carbenicillin[c]	Pseudomonas aeruginosa	25619	1	36–37.5	24 h	10	0.5
Cloxacillin	Staphylococcus aureus	29737	1	32–35	24 h	1	0.1
Colistimethate	Bordetella bronchiseptica	4617	1	32–35	24 h	10	0.1
Colistin	Bordetella bronchiseptica	4617	1	32–35	24 h	10	0.1
Dihydrostreptomycin	Bacillus subtilis	6633	32	32–35	5 days	5	As required
Erythromycin	Micrococcus luteus	9341	1	32–35	24 h	11	1.5
Gentamicin	Staphylococcus epidermidis	12228	1	32–35	24 h	11	0.03
Nafcillin	Staphylococcus aureus	29737	1	32–35	24 h	1	0.3
Neomycin	Staphylococcus epidermidis	12228	1	32–35	24 h	11	0.4
Novobiocin	Staphylococcus epidermidis	12228	1	32–35	24 h	1	4.0
Nystatin	Saccharomyces cerevisiae	2601	19	29–31	48 h	19	1.0
Paromomycin	Staphylococcus epidermidis	12228	1	32–35	24 h	11	2.0
Penicillin G	Staphylococcus aureus	29737	1	32–35	24 h	1	1.0
Polymyxin B	Bordetella bronchiseptica	4617	1	32–35	24 h	10	0.1
Sisomicin	Staphylococcus epidermidis	12228	1	32–35	24 h	11	0.03
Vancomycin	Bacillus subtilis	6633	32	32–35	5 days	8	As required

American Type Culture Collection, 10801 University Boulevard, Manassas VA 20110-2209 (http://www.atcc.org)
See Media and Solutions, Media.
Use 0.5 mL of a 1:25 dilution of the stock suspension/100 mL of Medium 10.

Analysis: Prepare the base layer for the required number of assay Petri plates, using the medium and volume shown in Table 51.4. Allow it to harden into a smooth base layer of uniform depth. Prepare the appropriate amount of seed layer inoculum (Table 51.5) as directed for the given antibiotic (Table 51.3) with any adjustments made based on the preparatory trial analysis. Tilt the plate back and forth to spread the inoculum evenly over the base layer surface, and allow it to harden.

Table 51.4 Preparation of Base Layer for Analysis

Antibiotic	Medium[a]	Target Volume (mL)
Amphotericin B[b]	—	—
Bleomycin	35	10
Carbenicillin	9	21
Colistimethate	9	21
Colistin	9	21
Dihydrostreptomycin	5	21
Erythromycin	11	21
Gentamicin	11	21
Neomycin	11	21
Nystatin[b]	—	—
Paromomycin	11	21
Polymyxin B	9	21
Sisomicin	11	21
Vancomycin	8	10
All others	2	21

a See Media and Solutions, Media.
b No base layer is used.
[Note—The base layer may be warmed to facilitate a uniform seed layer.]

Table 51.5 Preparation of Seed Layer for Analysis

Antibiotic	Medium[a]	Target Volume (mL)
Amphotericin B	Refer to Table 3	8
Bleomycin		6
Nystatin		8
All others		4

a See Media and Solutions, Media.

Drop six assay cylinders on the inoculated surface from a height of 12 mm, using a mechanical guide or other device to ensure even spacing on a radius of 2.8 cm, and cover the plates to avoid contamination. Fill the six cylinders on each plate with dilutions of antibiotic containing the test levels (S1–S5 and U3) specified in the following paragraph. Incubate the plates as specified in Table 51.6 for 16–18 h, and remove the cylinders. Measure and record the diameter of each zone of growth inhibition to the nearest 0.1 mm.

Table 51.6 Incubation temperature of analysis plates

Antibiotic	Incubation Temperature (ºC)
Amphotericin B	29–31
Carbenicillin	36–37.5
Colistimethate	36–37.5
Colistin	36–37.5
Dihydrostreptomycin	36–37.5
Gentamicin	36–37.5
Neomycin	36–37.5
Novobiocin	34–36
Nystatin	29–31
Paromomycin	36–37.5
Polymyxin B	36–37.5
Sisomicin	36–37.5
Vancomycin	36–37.5
All others	32–35

The standards (S1–S5) and a single test level of the sample (U3) corresponding to S3 of the standard curve, as defined in Standard solutions and Sample solutions will be used in the assay. For deriving the standard curve, fill alternate cylinders on each of three plates with the median test dilution (S3) of the standard and each of the remaining nine cylinders with one of the other four test dilutions of the standard. Repeat the process for the three test dilutions of the standard. For the sample, fill alternate cylinders on each of three plates with the median test dilution of the standard (S3), and fill the remaining nine cylinders with the corresponding test dilution (U3) of the sample.

Turbidimetric Method

Temperature control: Use appropriately qualified and calibrated equipment to obtain the temperature ranges specified in Table 51.8. [Note—Temperature control can be achieved using either circulating air or water. The greater heat capacity of water lends it some advantage over circulating air.]

Spectrophotometer: Measuring absorbance or transmittance within a fairly narrow frequency band requires a suitable spectrophotometer in which the wavelength can be varied or restricted by use of 580-nm or 530-nm filters. Alternatively, a variable-wavelength spectrophotometer can be used and set to a wavelength of 580 nm or 530 nm.

The instrument may be modified as follows:

1. To accept the tube in which incubation takes place (see Apparatus below)
2. To accept a modified cell fitted with a drain that facilitates rapid change of contents
3. To contain a flow cell for a continuous flow through analysis

Autozero the instrument with clear, uninoculated broth prepared as specified for the particular antibiotic, including the same amount of test dilution (including formaldehyde if specified) as found in each sample.

Either absorbance or transmittance can be measured while preparing inocula.

Apparatus: Glass or plastic test tubes, e.g., 16 × 125 mm or 18 × 150 mm. [Note—Use tubes that are relatively uniform in length, diameter, and thickness and substantially free from surface blemishes and scratches. In the spectrophotometer, use matched tubes that are free from scratches or blemishes. Clean tubes thoroughly to remove all antibiotic residues and traces of cleaning solution. Sterilize tubes before use.]

Standard solutions: To prepare a stock solution, dissolve a quantity of the USP Reference Standard of a given antibiotic or the entire contents of a vial of USP Reference Standard, where appropriate, in the solvent specified in Table 51.7, and dilute to the required concentration. Store at 2° –8°, and use within the period indicated. On the day of the assay, prepare from the stock solution five or more test dilutions, the successive solutions increasing stepwise in concentration, usually in the ratio of 1:1.25. [Note—It may be necessary to use smaller ratios for the successive dilutions from the stock solution for the turbidimetric assay]. Use the final diluent specified such that the median level of the standard (S3) has the concentration suggested in Table 51.7.

Sample solutions: Assign an assumed potency per unit weight or volume to the unknown, and on the day of the assay prepare a stock solution in the same manner specified for the USP Reference Standard (Table 51.7). Dilute the sample stock solution in the specified final diluent at a nominal concentration equal to the median concentration of the standard (S3) as specified in Table 51.7.

Table 51.7 Preparation of standard and sample solutions

Antibiotic	Stock Solution					Test Dilution	
	Initial Solvent	Initial Concentration	Further Diluent	Final Stock Concentration	Use Within	Final Diluent	Median Concentration (S3)[a]
Capreomycin	Water	—	—	1 mg/mL	7 days	Water	100 µg/mL
Chloramphenicol	Alcohol	10 mg/mL	Water	1 mg/mL	30 days	Water	2.5 µg/mL
Chlortetracycline	0.01 N hydrochloric acid	—	—	1 mg/mL	4 days	Water	0.06 µg/mL
Dihydrostreptomycin[b]	Water	—	—	1 mg/mL	30 days	Water	30 µg/mL
Gramicidin	Alcohol	—	—	1 mg/mL	30 days	Alcohol	0.04 µg/mL
Neomycin[b,d]	B.3[c]	—	—	100 µg/mL	14 days	B.3[c]	1.0 µg/mL
Oxytetracycline	0.1 N hydrochloric acid	—	—	1 mg/mL	4 days	Water	0.24 µg/mL
Tetracycline	0.1 N hydrochloric acid	—	—	1 mg/mL	1 day	Water	0.24 µg/mL
Thiostrepton	Dimethyl sulfoxide	—	—	1 U/mL	Same day	Dimethyl sulfoxide	0.80 U/mL
Troleandomycin	Isopropyl alcohol and water (4:1)	—	—	1 mg/mL	Same day	Water	25 µg/mL
Tylosin	Methanol	10 mg/mL	B.16[c]	1 mg/mL	30 days	Methanol and B.3[c] (1:1)	4 µg/mL

µg in this column refers to µg of activity.

The cylinder-plate assay can be used as an alternative procedure.

The letter B refers to buffer. See Media and Solutions, Buffers for a description of each buffer listed in this table.

Dilute the 100-µg/mL stock solution with Buffer B.3 to obtain a solution having a concentration equivalent to 25 µg/mL of neomycin. To separate 50-mL volumetric flasks add 1.39, 1.67, 2.00, 2.40, and 2.88 mL of this solution. Add 5.0 mL of 0.01 N hydrochloric acid to each flask, dilute with Buffer B.3 to volume, and mix to obtain solutions having concentrations of 0.69, 0.83, 1.0, 1.2, and 1.44 µg/mL of neomycin. Use these solutions to prepare the standard response line.

Inocula: Suspend the test organism from a freshly grown slant or culture in 3 mL of sterile saline TS. Glass beads can be used to facilitate the suspension. Enterococcus hirae (ATCC 10541) and Staphylococcus aureus (ATCC 9144) are grown in a liquid medium, not on agar. Spread the saline suspension onto the surface of two or more agar plates (covering the entire surface) or onto the surface of a Roux bottle containing 250 mL of the specified medium (see Table 51.8). Incubate at the time and temperature specified in Table 51.8, or until growth is apparent.

After incubation, harvest the organism from the plates or Roux bottle with approximately 50 mL of sterile saline TS, using a sterile bent glass rod or sterile glass beads. Pipet the suspension into a sterile glass bottle. This is the harvest suspension.

Determine during method verification the quantity of harvest suspension that will be used as the inoculum, starting with the volume suggested in Table 51.8. Prepare also an extra S3 as a test of growth. Incubate the trial tests for the times indicated in Table 51.11. Adjust the quantity of inoculum daily, if necessary, to obtain the optimum concentration–response relationship from the amount of growth of the test organism in the assay tubes. At the completion of the specified incubation periods, tubes containing the median concentration of the standard should have absorbance values as specified in Table 51.9. Determine the exact duration of incubation by observing the growth in the reference concentration (median concentration) of the standard (S3).

Table 51.8 Incubation Condition of Test Organism

Antibiotic	Test Organism	ATCC[a] Number	Incubation Conditions			Suggested Inoculum Composition	
			Medium[b]	Tempe-rature (°)	Time	Medium[b]	Amount (mL/100 mL)
Capreomycin	*Klebsiella pneumoniae*	10031	1	36–37.5	16–24 h	3	0.05
Chloramphenicol	*Escherichia coli*	10536	1	32–35	24 h	3	0.7
Chlortetracycline	*Staphylococcus aureus*	29737	1	32–35	24 h	3	0.1
Dihydrostreptomycin	*Klebsiella pneumoniae*	10031	1	36–37.5	16–24 h	3	0.1
Gramicidin	*Enterococcus hirae*	10541	3	36–37.5	16–18 h	3	1.0
Neomycin	*Klebsiella pneumoniae*	10031	1	36–37.5	16–24 h	39	2
Oxytetracycline	*Staphylococcus aureus*	29737	1	32–35	24 h	3	0.1

Table 51.8 *Contd...*

Antibiotic	Test Organism	ATCC[a] Number	Incubation Conditions			Suggested Inoculum Composition	
			Medium[b]	Tempe-rature (°)	Time	Medium[b]	Amount (mL/100 mL)
Tetracycline	*Staphylococc us aureus*	29737	1	32–35	24 h	3	0.1
Thiostrepton	*Enterococcus hirae*	10541	40	36–37.5	18–24 h	41	0.2
Troleandomycin	*Klebsiella pneumoniae*	10031	1	36–37.5	16–24 h	3	0.1
Tylosin	*Staphylococc us aureus*	9144	3	35–39	16–18 h	39	2–3

a American Type Culture Collection, 10801 University Boulevard, Manassas VA 20110-2209 (http://www.atcc.org)
b See Media and Solutions, Media.

Table 51.9 Absorbance values of standards

Antibiotic	Absorbance, NLT (a.u.)
Capreomycin	0.4
Chlortetracycline	0.35
Gramicidin	0.35
Tetracycline	0.35
All others	0.3

Analysis: On the day of the assay, prepare the necessary concentration of antibiotic by dilution of stock solutions of the standard and of each sample as specified under Standard solutions and Sample solutions. Prepare five test levels, each in triplicate, of the standard (S1–S5) and a single test level (U3), also in triplicate, of up to 20 samples corresponding to S3 (median concentration) of the standard.

Table 51.10 Preparation of antibiotic dilutions

Antibiotic	Volume of Test Dilution (mL)	Volume of Inoculum (mL)
Gramicidin	0.10	9.0
Thiostrepton	0.10	10.0
Tylosin	0.10	9.0
All others	1.0	9.0

Place the tubes in test tube racks or other carriers. Include in each rack 1–2 control tubes containing 1 mL of the inoculum medium (see Table 51.8) but no antibiotic. Add the volumes of the standard and sample test dilutions as indicated in Table 51.10. Randomly distribute one complete set, including the controls, in a tube rack. Add the volume of inoculum specified in Table 51.10 to each tube in the rack in turn, and place the completed rack immediately in an incubator or a water bath maintained at the temperature specified in Table 51.8 and for the time specified in Table 51.11.

Table 51.11 Incubation time of antibiotics

Antibiotic	Incubation Time (h)
Capreomycin	3–4
Chloramphenicol	3–4
Cycloserine	3–4
Dihydrostreptomycin	3–4
Streptomycin	3–4
Troleandomycin	3–4
Tylosin	3–5
All others	4–5

After incubation, immediately inhibit the growth of the organism by adding 0.5 mL of dilute formaldehyde to each tube, except for tylosin. For tylosin, heat the rack in a water bath at 80 ºC –90 ºC for 2–6 min or in a steam bath for 5–10 min, and bring to room temperature. Read absorbance or transmittance at 530 or 580 nm, analyzing one rack at a time.

Media and Solutions

The media required for the preparation of test organism inocula are made from the ingredients listed herein. Minor modifications of the individual ingredients are acceptable; and reconstituted dehydrated media can be substituted, provided that the resulting media possess equal or better growth-promoting properties and give a similar standard curve response.

Media: Dissolve the ingredients in water to make 1 L, and adjust the solutions with either 1 N sodium hydroxide or 1 N hydrochloric acid as required, so that after steam sterilization the pH is as specified.

Medium 1

Peptone	6.0 g
Pancreatic digest of casein	4.0 g
Yeast extract	3.0 g
Beef extract	1.5 g
Dextrose	1.0 g
Agar	15.0 g
Water	1000 mL
pH after sterilization	6.6 ± 0.1

Medium 2

Peptone	6.0 g
Yeast extract	3.0 g
Beef extract	1.5 g
Agar	15.0 g
Water	1000 mL
pH after sterilization	6.6 ± 0.1

Medium 3

Peptone	5.0 g
Yeast extract	1.5 g
Beef extract	1.5 g
Sodium chloride	3.5 g
Dextrose	1.0 g
Dibasic potassium phosphate	3.68 g
Monobasic potassium phosphate	1.32 g
Water	1000 mL
pH after sterilization	7.0 ± 0.05

Medium 4

Peptone	6.0 g
Yeast extract	3.0 g
Beef extract	1.5 g
Dextrose	1.0 g
Agar	15.0 g
Water	1000 mL
pH after sterilization	6.6 ± 0.1

Medium 5

Peptone	6.0 g
Yeast extract	3.0 g
Beef extract	1.5 g
Agar	15.0 g
Water	1000 mL
pH after sterilization	7.9 ± 0.1

Medium 8

Peptone	6.0 g
Yeast extract	3.0 g
Beef extract	1.5 g
Agar	15.0 g
Water	1000 mL
pH after sterilization	5.9 ± 0.1

Medium 9

Pancreatic digest of casein	17.0 g
Papaic digest of soybean	3.0 g
Sodium chloride	5.0 g
Dibasic potassium phosphate	2.5 g
Dextrose	2.5 g
Agar	20.0 g
Water	1000 mL
pH after sterilization	7.2 ± 0.1

Medium 10

Pancreatic digest of casein	17.0 g
Papaic digest of soybean	3.0 g
Sodium chloride	5.0 g
Dibasic potassium phosphate	2.5 g
Dextrose	2.5 g
Agar	12.0 g
Water	1000 mL
Polysorbate 80 (added after boiling the medium to dissolve the agar)	10 mL
pH after sterilization	7.2 ± 0.1

Medium 11

Peptone	6.0 g
Pancreatic digest of casein	4.0 g
Yeast extract	3.0 g
Beef extract	1.5 g
Dextrose	1.0 g
Agar	15.0 g
Water	1000 mL
pH after sterilization	8.3 ± 0.1

Medium 13

Peptone	10.0 g
Dextrose	20.0 g
Water	1000 mL
pH after sterilization	5.6 ± 0.1

Medium 19

Peptone	9.4 g
Yeast extract	4.7 g
Beef extract	2.4 g
Sodium chloride	10.0 g
Dextrose	10.0 g
Agar	23.5 g
Water	1000 mL
pH after sterilization	6.1 ± 0.1

Medium 32

Peptone	6.0 g
Pancreatic digest of casein	4.0 g
Yeast extract	3.0 g
Beef extract	1.5 g
Manganese sulfate	0.3 g
Dextrose	1.0 g
Agar	15.0 g
Water	1000 mL
pH after sterilization	6.6 ± 0.1

Medium 34

Glycerol	10.0 g
Peptone	10.0 g
Beef extract	10.0 g
Sodium chloride	3.0 g
Water	1000 mL
pH after sterilization	7.0 ± 0.1

Medium 35

Glycerol	10.0 g
Peptone	10.0 g
Beef extract	10.0 g
Sodium chloride	3.0 g
Agar	17.0 g
Water	1000 mL
pH after sterilization	7.0 ± 0.1

Medium 36

Pancreatic digest of casein	15.0 g
Papaic digest of soybean	5.0 g
Sodium chloride	5.0 g
Agar	15.0 g
Water	1000 mL
pH after sterilization	7.3 ± 0.1

Medium 39

Peptone	5.0 g
Yeast extract	1.5 g
Beef extract	1.5 g
Sodium chloride	3.5 g
Dextrose	1.0 g
Dibasic potassium phosphate	3.68 g
Monobasic potassium phosphate	1.32 g
Water	1000 mL
pH after sterilization	7.9 ± 0.1

Medium 40

Yeast extract	20.0 g
Polypeptone	5.0 g
Dextrose	10.0 g
Monobasic potassium phosphate	2.0 g
Polysorbate 80	0.1 g
Agar	10.0 g
Water	1000 mL
pH after sterilization	6.7 ± 0.2

Medium 41

Pancreatic digest of casein	9.0 g
Dextrose	20.0 g
Yeast extract	5.0 g
Sodium citrate	10.0 g
Monobasic potassium phosphate	1.0 g
Dibasic potassium phosphate	1.0 g
Water	1000 mL
pH after sterilization	6.8 ± 0.1

Solutions

Buffers: Prepare as directed in Table 51.12, or by other suitable means. The buffers are sterilized after preparation; the pH specified in each case is the pH after sterilization.

Table 51.12 Preparation of buffers

Buffer	Concentration of Dibasic Potassium Phosphate (g/L)	Concentration of Monobasic Potassium Phosphate (g/L)	Volume of 10 N Potassium Hydroxide (mL)	pH after Sterilization[a]
Buffer B.1 (1%, pH 6.0)	2	8	—	6.0 ± 0.05
Buffer B.3 (0.1 M, pH 8.0)	16.73	0.523	—	8.0 ± 0.1
Buffer B.4 (0.1 M, pH 4.5)	—	13.61	—	4.5 ± 0.05
Buffer B.6 (10%, pH 6.0)	20	80	—	6.0 ± 0.05

Table 51.12 *Contd...*

Buffer	Concentration of Dibasic Potassium Phosphate (g/L)	Concentration of Monobasic Potassium Phosphate (g/L)	Volume of 10 N Potassium Hydroxide (mL)	pH after Sterilization[a]
Buffer B.10 (0.2 M, pH 10.5)	35	—	2	10.5 ± 0.1
Buffer B.16 (0.1 M, pH 7.0)	13.6	4	—	7.0 ± 0.2

a Adjust the pH with 18 N phosphoric acid or 10 N potassium hydroxide.

Other solutions: See Reagents, Indicators, and Solutions.

Water: Use Purified Water.

Saline: Use saline TS.

Dilute formaldehyde: Formaldehyde solution and water (1:3)

Calculations

Introduction: Antibiotic potency is calculated by interpolation from a standard curve using a log-transformed straight-line method with a least-squares fitting procedure (see below for calculation details). The analyst must consider three essential concepts in interpreting antibiotic potency results:

1. Biological concentration–response relationships generally are not linear. The antibiotic potency method allows fitting the data to a straight line by evaluating a narrow concentration range where the results approach linearity. The assay results can be considered valid only if the computed potency is 80%–125% of that assumed in preparing the sample stock solution. When the calculated potency value falls outside 80%–125%, the result for the sample may fall outside the narrow concentration range where linearity has been established. In such a case, adjust the assumed potency of the sample accordingly, and repeat the assay to obtain a valid result.

2. The most effective means of reducing the variability of the reportable value (the geometric mean potency across runs and replicates) is through independent runs of the assay procedure. The combined result of a series of smaller, independent assays spread over a number of days is a more reliable estimate of potency than that from a single large assay with the same total number of plates or tubes. Three or more independent assays are required for antibiotic potency determinations.

3. The number of assays needed in order to obtain a reliable estimate of antibiotic potency depends on the required specification range and the assay variability. The confidence limit calculation described below is determined from several estimated log potencies that are approximately equal in precision. If the value calculated for the width of the confidence interval, W, is too wide, no useful decision can be made about whether the potency meets its specification.

The laboratory should predetermine in its standard operating procedures a maximum acceptable value for the confidence interval width. This maximum value should be determined during development and confirmed during validation or verification. If the calculated confidence interval width exceeds this limit, the analyst must perform additional independent potency determinations to meet the limit requirement. Note that the decision to perform additional determinations does not depend on the estimated potency but only on the uncertainty in that estimate as determined by the confidence interval width. Assay variability has a greater impact on the calculated confidence limit than does the number of independent potency determinations. As a result, the analyst should first consider decreasing variability to the extent possible before conducting potency determinations.

The following sections describe the calculations for determining antibiotic potency as well as for performing the confidence limit calculation. Methods for calculating standard error are also shown in order to allow estimates of assay variance. Where logarithms are used, any base log is acceptable. Appendix 1 provides formulas for hand calculations applicable when the concentrations are equally spaced in the log scale. Alternative statistical methods may be used if appropriately validated.

Cylinder-plate assay: This section details analysis of the sample data and determination of the potency of an unknown, using the cylinder-plate assay.

Sample data: Table 51.13 shows the data from one assay that will be used as an example throughout this section. For each of the 12 plates, zones 1, 3, and 5 are the reference concentration and the other three zones are for one of the other four concentrations, as shown. Other columns are needed for calculations and are explained below.

Step 1: Perform initial calculations and variability suitability check.

For each set of three plates, average the nine reference values and average the nine standard values.

Example (see Table 51.13)

$$15.867 = X(16.1, 15.6, ..., 15.8)$$

$$14.167 = X(14.6, 14.1, ..., 14.8)$$

For each set of three plates determine the standard deviation of the nine reference values and the standard deviation of the nine standard values. For each standard deviation, determine the corresponding relative standard deviation.

Example (see Table 51.13)

$$0.200 = \sigma(16.1, ..., 15.8)$$

$$1.3\% = (0.200/15.867) \times 100$$

$$0.324 = \sigma(14.6, ..., 14.1)$$

$$2.3\% = (0.324/14.167) \times 100$$

For a variability suitability criterion, each laboratory should determine a maximum acceptable value for the relative standard deviation. If any of the eight relative standard deviations (four for the reference and four for the standard) exceed this predetermined maximum, the assay data are not suitable and should be discarded. [Note—The suggested limit for relative standard deviation is NMT 10%.]

Step 2: Perform a plate-to-plate variation correction.

This correction is applied to convert the average zone measurement obtained for each concentration to the value it would be if the average reference concentration measurement for that set of three replicate plates were the same as the value of the correction point:

$$XC = XS - (XR - P)$$

XC = corrected standard mean

XS = original standard mean

XR = reference mean

P = correction point

Example: For the first set of three plates in Table 51.13 (S1), the correction is:

$$14.022 = 14.167 - (15.867 - 15.722) = 14.167 - 0.145$$

Table 51.13 Sample data (Cylinder-Plate Assay)

Standard	Concentration (U/mL)	Plate replicate	Reference (S3)						Sample						Corrected Mean (mm)
			Zone 1 (mm)	Zone 3 (mm)	Zone 5 (mm)	Mean (mm)	SD	%RSD	Zone 2 (mm)	Zone 4 (mm)	Zone 6 (mm)	Mean (mm)	SD	%RSD	
S1	3.20	1	16.1	15.6	15.8	15.867	0.200	1.3	14.6	14.1	13.5	14.167	0.324	2.3	14.022
		2	16.0	15.9	16.2				14.5	14.1	14.4				
		3	15.7	15.7	15.8				14.0	14.2	14.1				
S2	4.00	1	15.8	15.6	15.5	15.567	0.158	1.0	14.7	15.1	14.8	14.833	0.265	1.8	14.989
		2	15.7	15.5	15.6				14.7	14.9	15.2				
		3	15.7	15.4	15.3				14.8	15.0	14.3				
S4	6.25	1	15.6	15.8	16.0	15.789	0.169	1.1	16.6	16.8	16.3	16.578	0.233	1.4	16.511
		2	15.8	15.6	15.7				16.6	16.5	16.2				
		3	16.1	15.7	15.8				16.9	16.5	16.8				
S5	7.8125	1	15.6	15.6	15.5	15.667	0.141	0.9	17.3	17.0	17.0	17.167	0.224	1.3	17.222
		2	15.6	15.7	15.5				17.3	17.4	17.2				
		3	15.9	15.8	15.8				17.3	17.3	16.7				
						15.722[a]									
U3	unknown	1	15.7	15.8	15.7	15.678	0.179	1.1	15.3	15.8	15.7	15.478	0.307	2.0	15.522
		2	15.9	15.7	15.7				15.8	15.8	15.5				
		3	15.5	15.8	15.3				15.2	15.1	15.1				

a This is the value of the overall reference mean, referred to as the "correction point" below.

Step 3: Determine the standard curve line.

Generate the standard curve line by plotting the corrected zone measurements versus the log of the standard concentration values. Calculate the equation of the standard curve line by performing a standard unweighted linear regression on these values, using appropriate software or the manual calculations of Appendix 1. [Note—Use either the natural log or the base 10 log to plot the standard curve and determine the regression equation; both provide the same final test result.] Each laboratory should determine a minimum value of the coefficient of determination (%R2) for an acceptable regression. The regression is acceptable only if they obtained %R2 exceeds this predetermined value. [Note—The suggested limit for the percentage coefficient of determination is NLT 95%.]

Example: Table 51.14 summarizes the portion of Table 51.13 needed for this part of the calculation.

Table 51.14 Corrected zone measurements

Standard Set	Corrected Zone Measurements (mm)	Concentration (U/mL)
S1	14.022	3.2
S2	14.989	4.0
Reference (S3)	15.722	5
S4	16.511	6.25
S5	17.222	7.8125

Linear regression results

Standard curve line:

$$Z = [3.551 \times \ln(C)] + 9.978$$

Z = corrected zone measurement

C = concentration

%R2 = 99.7

Sample potency determination: To estimate the potency of the unknown sample, average the zone measurements of the standard and the zone measurements of the sample on the three plates used. Correct for plate-to-plate variation using the correction point determined above to obtain a corrected average for the unknown, U. [Note—An acceptable alternative to using the correction point is to correct using the value on the estimated regression line corresponding to the log concentration of S3]. Use the corrected average zone measurement in the equation of the standard curve line to determine the log concentration of the sample, LU, by:

$$LU = (U - a)/b$$

a = intercept of the regression line

b = slope of the regression line

To obtain the potency of the unknown, take the antilog of LU and multiply the result by any applicable dilution factor. This value can also be expressed as a percentage of the reference concentration value.

Example: Corrected sample zone measurement (Table 51.13) = 15.522

Natural log of the sample concentration:

$$LU = (15.522 - 9.978)/3.551 = 1.561$$

Sample concentration:

$$CU = e1.561 = 4.765$$

Percentage of reference concentration:

$$Result = (4.765/5.000) \times 100 = 95.3\%$$

Turbidimetric assay: This section details analysis of the sample data and determination of the potency of an unknown using the turbidimetric assay. The method assumes that the tubes are randomly distributed within the heat block or other temperature control device. If the device has a temperature profile that is not uniform, a randomized blocks design is preferred. In such a design, the rack is divided into areas (blocks) of relatively uniform temperature and at least one tube of each Standard concentration and of each unknown is placed in each area. The data analysis of a randomized block design is different from the following.

Sample data: Table 51.15 shows the data from one assay that will be used for an example throughout this section. Other columns are needed for calculations and are explained below.

Table 51.15 Sample Data (Turbidimetric Assay)

Standard	Concentration (μg/mL)	Replicate	Absorbance (a.u.)	Average (a.u.)	Standard Deviation
S1	64	1	0.8545	0.8487	0.0062
		2	0.8422		
		3	0.8495		
S2	80	1	0.8142	0.8269	0.0125
		2	0.8273		
		3	0.8392		
S3	100	1	0.6284	0.6931	0.0640
		2	0.6947		
		3	0.7563		
S4	125	1	0.6933	0.6827	0.0119
		2	0.6850		
		3	0.6699		
S5	156	1	0.5299	0.5465	0.0272
		2	0.5779		
		3	0.5316		
U3	unknown	1	0.7130	0.7430	0.0460
		2	0.7960		
		3	0.7201		

Step 1: Perform initial calculations and variability suitability check.

For each concentration (including the sample), average the three absorbance values.

Example: See S1 in Table 51.15.

$$0.8487 = X(0.8545, 0.8422, 0.8495)$$

For each concentration, determine the standard deviation of the three readings and a combined standard deviation for all the concentrations.

Example: See S1 in Table 51.15.

$$0.0125 = SD(0.8545, 0.8422, 0.8495)$$

The combined value is calculated by taking the square root of the average of the five variances:

$$0.0325 = \{[(0.0062)2 + (0.0125)2 + (0.0640)2 + (0.0119)2 + (0.0272)2]/5\}1/2$$

For a variability suitability criterion, each laboratory should determine a maximum acceptable combined standard deviation. If the combined standard deviation exceeds this predetermined maximum, the assay data are not suitable and should be discarded. [Note—The suggested limit for the combined standard deviation is NMT 10% of the average absorbance value across the five concentrations] If the number of replicates per concentration is atleast five, then a relative standard deviation can be computed for each concentration after checking for outliers and compared to a maximum acceptable relative standard deviation. [Note—The suggested limit for the relative standard deviation is NMT 10%].

Step 2: Determine the standard curve line.

Generate the standard curve line by plotting the average absorbance values versus the log of the standard concentration values. Calculate the equation of the standard curve line by performing an unweighted linear regression on these values using appropriate software or the manual calculations of Appendix 1. [Note—Use either the natural log or the base 10 log to plot the standard curve and determine the regression equation; both provide the same final test result]. Each laboratory should determine a minimum value of the percentage coefficient of determination (%R2) for an acceptable regression. The regression is acceptable only if the %R2 value obtained exceeds this predetermined value. [Note—The suggested limit for the percentage coefficient of determination is NLT 90%].

Example: Table 51.16 summarizes the portion of Table 15 needed for this part of the calculation.

Table 51.16 Determination of standard curve line

Set of Standards	Average Absorbance Values (a.u.)	Concentration (µg/mL)
S1	0.8487	64
S2	0.8269	80
S3	0.6931	100
S4	0.6827	125
S5	0.5465	156

Linear regression results

Standard curve line:

Absorbance = 2.2665 – [0.7735 × $\log_{10}$ (concentration)]

%R2 = 93.0%

Sample potency determination: To estimate the potency of the unknown sample, average the three absorbance measurements to obtain an average for the unknown, U. Use this average measurement in the equation of the standard curve line to determine the log concentration of the unknown sample, LU, by:

$$LU = (U - a)/b$$

a = intercept of the regression line

b = slope of the regression line

To obtain the potency of the unknown, take the antilog of LU and multiply the result by any applicable dilution factor. This value can also be expressed as a percentage of the reference concentration value.

Example: Average sample absorbance (Table 51.15) = 0.7430.

$$\log 10(CU) = (0.7430 - 2.2665)/(-0.7735) = 1.9696$$

$$CU = 101.9696 = 93.2$$

Percentage of reference concentration = (93.2/100.0) × 100 = 93.2%

CU = concentration of the sample

Confidence limits and combination of assays calculations: Because of interassay variability, three or more independent determinations are required for a reliable estimate of the sample potency. For each independent determination, start with separately prepared stock solutions and test dilutions of both the Standard and the sample, and repeat the assay of a given sample on a different day.

Given a set of atleast three determinations of the unknown potency, use the method of Appendix 2 to check for any outlier values. This determination should be done in the log scale.

To obtain a combined estimate of the unknown potency, calculate the average, M, and the standard deviation of the accepted log potencies. [Note—Use either the natural log or the base 10 log.] Determine the confidence interval for the potency as follows:

$$\text{antilog}[M - t(0.05, N - 1) \times SD/\sqrt{N}]$$

$$\text{antilog}[M + t(0.05, N - 1) \times SD/\sqrt{N}]$$

M = average

SD = standard deviation

N = number of assays

t (0.05, N – 1) = the two-sided 5% point of a Student's t-distribution with N – 1 degrees of freedom

Note: The t value is available in spreadsheets, statistics texts, and statistics software.

$$W = \text{antilog } \{[t(0.05, N - 1) \times SD / \sqrt{N}]\}$$

W = half-width of the confidence interval

Compare the half-width of the confidence interval to a predetermined maximum acceptable value. If the half-width is larger than the acceptance limit, continue with additional assays.

Example: Suppose the sample is assayed four times, with potency results in the natural log scale of 1.561, 1.444, 1.517, and 1.535. Then:

$$N = 4$$

$$M = X(1.561, 1.444, 1.517, 1.535) = 1.514$$

$$SD = \sigma(1.561, 1.444, 1.517, 1.535) = 0.050$$

$$t = 3.182$$

The confidence interval in the log scale is

$$1.514 \pm (3.182 \times 0.050/\sqrt{4}) = (1.434, 1.594)$$

Taking antilogs, the estimated potency is

$$e1.514 = 4.546$$

With a 95% confidence interval for the potency of e1.434, e 1.594 = (4.197, 4.924).

The confidence interval half-width to compare to an acceptance value is the ratio 4.924/4.546 = 1.083.

Appendix 1. Formulas for Manual Calculations of Regression and Sample Concentration

If the concentrations are equally spaced in the logarithmic scale, the calculations can be performed using the following formula. Let:

Sk = mean corrected zone measurement (cylinder-plate assay) or average absorbance value (turbidimetric assay) for standard set k

k = 1, 2, 3, 4, 5

S = mean of the five Sk values

Lk = logarithm of the kth concentration. [Note—Use either the natural log or the base 10 log. Slope of the regression line is calculated by:]

$$b = (Y_{high} - Y_{low})/(X_{high} - X_{low})$$

$$Y_{high} = 1/5(3S5 + 2S4 + S3 - S1)$$

$$Y_{low} = 1/5(3S1 + 2S2 + S3 - S5)$$

$$Xhigh = L5$$

$$Xlow = L1$$

Combine and simplify to:

$$b = (4S5 + 2S4 - 2S2 - 4S1)/[5(L5 - L1)]$$

The log of the concentration of the sample is found using:

$$LU = Lreference + [(U - S)/b]$$

For example, using the data for the cylinder-plate assay in Table 51.13 and natural logarithms:

$$b = [(4 \times 17.222) + (2 \times 16.511) - (2 \times 14.989) -$$

$$(4 \times 14.020)]/\{5[\ln(7.81)] - \ln(3.2)\} = 3.551$$

$$S = (14.020 + 14.989 + 15.722 + 16.511 + 17.222)/5 = 15.693$$

Natural log of sample concentration =

$$\ln(5) + [(15.522 - 15.693)/3.551] = 1.561$$

Sample concentration = e1.561 = 4.765

Appendix 2. Procedure for Checking for Outliers; Rejection of Outlying or Aberrant Measurements

A measurement that is clearly questionable because of a failure in the assay procedure should be rejected, whether it is discovered during the measuring or tabulation procedure. The arbitrary rejection or retention of an apparently aberrant measurement can be a serious source of bias. In general, the rejection of measurements solely on the basis of their relative magnitudes is a procedure that should be used sparingly.

Each suspected potency measurement, or outlier, may be tested against the following criterion. This criterion is based on the variation within a single group of supposedly equivalent measurements from a normal distribution. On average, it will reject a valid observation once in 25 trials or once in 50 trials. Designate the measurements in order of magnitude from y1 to yN, where y1 is the candidate outlier, and N is the number of measurements in the group. Compute the relative gap by using Table A2-1, Test for Outlier Measurements, and the formulas below:

When N = 3 to 7:

$$G1 = (y2 - y1)/(yN - y1)$$

When N = 8 to 10:

$$G2 = (y2 - y1)/(yN - 1 - y1)$$

When N = 11 to 13:

$$G3 = (y3 - y1)/(yN - 1 - y1)$$

If G1, G2, or G3, as appropriate, exceeds the critical value in Table A2-1, Test for Outlier Measurements, for the observed N, there is a statistical basis for omitting the outlier measurement(s).

Table A2-1 Test for Outlier Measurements

In samples from a normal population, gaps equal to or larger than the following values of G1, G2, and G3 occur with a probability P = 0.01, when outlier measurements can occur only at one end; or with P = 0.02, when they may occur at either end.				
N	3	4	5	6	7
G1	0.987	0.889	0.781	0.698	0.637
N	8	9	10		
G2	0.681	0.634	0.597		
N	11	12	13		
G3	0.674	0.643	0.617		

Example: Estimated potencies of sample in log scale = 1.561, 1.444, 1.517, 1.535.

Check lowest potency for outlier:

$$G1 = (1.517 - 1.444)/(1.561 - 1.444) = 0.624 < 0.889$$

Therefore 1.444 is not an outlier.

Check highest potency for outlier:

$$G1 = (1.561 - 1.535)/(1.561 - 1.444) = 0.222 < 0.889$$

Therefore 1.561 is not an outlier.

Outlier potencies should be marked as outlier values and excluded from the assay calculations. NMT one potency can be excluded as an outlier.

Printed in the USA
CPSIA information can be obtained
at www.ICGtesting.com
LVHW051109250724
786491LV00003B/23